How to
Understand and *Treat*
Your Child's Symptoms

How to
Understand and *Treat*
Your Child's Symptoms

Neil C. Henderson, M.D.

Parker Publishing Company, Inc.   *West Nyack, N.Y.*

© 1971, by

NEIL C. HENDERSON, M.D.

Library of Congress
Catalog Card Number: 76-150095

Printed in the United States of America
ISBN-0-13-435636-5
B & P

Dedication

This book is dedicated to my children, Paige and Walker, whom I love and enjoy. May I have the wisdom to guide them through the years so that we may still be good friends when they reach maturity.

How to
Understand and *Treat*
Your Child's Symptoms

The Purpose of This Book and How to Use It

I feel sure I needn't convince you that one of the most rewarding experiences life has to offer is the opportunity to be a parent. But, as the rewards of child raising are to many parents unparalleled, so also can the responsibilities be awesome.

It is a universally accepted principle that fear is a companion to love—fear of failure, fear of loss. In a mature person, fear takes the form of concern. Love needs no modification. A healthy blend of love and intelligent concern produces a satisfied and happy parent—not to mention a satisfied and happy child.

The difference between irrational fear and intelligent concern is the difference between ignorance and knowledgeability. Most occasions that give rise to concern for your child—especially a pre-school child—will concern his or her health.

All children get sick. Sickness is as much a part of childhood as teddy bears and bicycles. And yet, reassuringly, most children grow up to be healthy adults.

A child needs attention and intelligent care. Given this, he stands an excellent chance of never facing a truly serious crisis as far as his health is concerned. On a worldwide scale, a child's greatest danger lies in accidents and malnutrition.

The intelligent parent will devote some time and effort to learning about the diseases and maladies that are common to childhood. More especially, a parent whose child suffers a chronic malady should inform himself fully on the nature of the condition.

The purpose of this book is to enable parents to relax and enjoy their child in order that they may cope confidently with the health challenges of child raising.

This is not a book to be read chronologically from cover to cover. My intention has been to provide a handy and practical reference that parents may consult as specific questions and problems arise. It is my feeling that you will derive the greatest benefit by referring to the book constantly and re-reading individual sections when your child has a particular problem.

Most important, I hope I have provided a practical means in helping you differentiate between the simple, uncomplicated problems affecting your children (which can be handled adequately without consulting your physician) and the more serious problems which require the attention—perhaps the immediate attention— of a physician.

You will know what I mean when I say that one of a parent's very real problems is the question of when or whether to call the doctor. It is not generally a matter of money—more often it is a matter of not wanting to make a fool out of oneself. In theory it is easy to say when you have the slightest doubt "call the doctor and be on the safe side." When? At midnight? For a minor belly-ache? Can it wait until morning? Let's face it: you are a human being and so is your doctor. He is subject to irritability, perhaps brusqueness on occasion, and you are subject to embarrassment. The parent who habitually calls the doctor needlessly, eventually is likely to not call him when he should.

It has long been my feeling that it would be a great comfort to a parent to be able to quickly and conveniently familiarize himself —and often re-familiarize himself—with the salient points of a child's health problem immediately at hand. A parent so armed will know exactly when to ask his doctor for help.

The General Index at the end of the book is a key part of this, book. I have tried to anticipate every conceivable description of every symptom a child might have. I am pretty certain a parent won't have to try to consult too many terms before ascertaining what a child's condition may be. For example, you would be directed to the section on the common cold by looking under "C" for "common cold" or "*C*" for "cold, common" or, as a matter of fact, "*U*" for "upper respiratory infection."

Looking up specific symptoms such as "Sneezing"; "Mucous, green or yellow"; "Nasal Discharge"; "Nasal Obstruction" would also refer you to the "common cold." By looking up each symptom you will increase your accuracy of assessment of the possible common cause. A quick reference Index of Symptoms will be found at the beginning of the book for your added convenience.

Just as I have aimed for completeness in the indexing of the subject matter, I have striven for completeness in the subject matter itself. For example, under each contagious disease (each of which has been indexed under any name I have ever heard it called) you will find the following eight crucial factors necessary to the understanding of any contagious disease:

1. The *signs and symptoms*—how to recognize disease.
2. The *cause* of the disease.
3. The proper *treatment* of the disease.
4. The *incubation* period—the elapsed time between exposure and the development of symptoms.
5. The period of *communicability*—the period of time during which your child could pass the disease on to another person.
6. *School attendance*—the amount of time your child will be absent from school due to the contraction of a specific disease.
7. *Prevention*—steps that may be taken to diminish the chances that your child will get the disease in the first place.
8. *Complications*—ways to avoid secondary infection and how to recognize secondary symptoms that are commonly associated with a specific illness.

In this book, under the "Common Cold" alone, you will find fifteen helpful suggestions regarding treatment.

You will learn of the many effective medications available in the drugstore without a prescription. You will learn how to determine the proper specific dosages of these, and other, medications for your child.

15

With the aid of this book you will learn the difference between special formulas and regular milk—how to take temperatures and control high fever—how to recognize the development of complications from a common cold—how to differentiate between various types of rashes, etc.

Parents with specific problems will find innumerable suggestions —such as programs that may be implemented for the prevention of asthma attacks or recurrent rheumatic fever. You will find specific answers to questions such as this: Should I call the doctor now or wait 24 to 48 hours? May I give medication by myself? Is it safe to attend school? If exposed to a contagious disease, can my child be given medication to prevent it?

In sum and substance, this book is a collection of clinical insights gathered through my years of varied experiences as a pediatrician. I have tried to answer questions in the same manner as I would if you were sitting opposite me in my examination room. If anything, I have answered the questions more fully in the book than time pressure would ordinarily allow in the office, and I have answered all questions honestly and candidly with no attempt to minimize problems.

This book, however, is by no means meant to restrict treatment recommended by your physician. My objective is to help you become an expert parent—not an expert physician. I hope that this book will help you, as a parent, not only to assume more responsibility for yourself (which is important) but that, through your improved judgment, you will also be able to develop a better relationship with your family physician or pediatrician.

It is my greatest hope that the constant use of this book will bring you peace of mind through understanding your child's symptoms of sickness and what you may do at home about them.

NEIL C. HENDERSON, M.D.

ACKNOWLEDGMENTS

I am grateful to my close friend, DONALD G. WORDEN, Editor of the Worden Taped Reading Studies, for encouraging me to write this book. My mind has been stimulated by his acute analytical thinking. I also wish to thank my friends and colleagues who read this manuscript and contributed suggestions, particularly Jane Foltz and Dr. Marvin Rosenblatt. I also wish to thank Milton S. Henderson, my father, whose guidance and support enabled me to become a physician.

Table of Contents

Index of Symptoms

This index sets up in alphabetical order the important symptoms or first things a parent should look for regarding the usual illnesses of a child seen in a physician's office.

For example, under Anemia, you are referred to Iron Deficiency, and Sickle Cell Anemia, as they appear in this book. Although Anemia occurs with other illnesses discussed in this book, those illnesses are so rare and are associated with other major symptoms that they should not be of practical consideration to the lay reader.

By looking up more than one symptom regarding an illness, your chances of getting a more accurate assessment of the condition are greatly increased. For example, you are referred to Diabetes under the symptoms of Coma, Urination (increased), and Weight Loss.

Remember, information about many other disorders may be found by referring to the General Index at the back of the book.

20

22

26

A

ABSCESSES, BOILS, CARBUNCLES

An abscess is a localized collection of pus in the tissues of the body.

A boil is a painful inflammatory sore forming a central core caused by a microbic infection. It is also known as a furuncle.

A carbuncle is a circumscribed inflammation of the tissue resulting in sloughing and having a tendency to spread. It is more serious than a boil.

The classical signs of these infections are:

1. Heat
2. Swelling
3. Pain
4. Tenderness

Treatment consists of antibiotics, hot soaks and, if the lesion comes to a head, incision and drainage. This minor surgery procedure may be done in your physician's office. It is not painful. However, with early antibiotic therapy, these lesions are sometimes absorbed by the body without coming to a head. (See Hot Soaks.)

ACCIDENTAL SWALLOWING OF CORROSIVE SUBSTANCES —CHEMICAL INJURIES

The stomach and esophagus are frequently affected by chemical injuries due to the accidental ingestion of poisons. Strong alkalies are sometimes taken in solutions by children because of their milk-like appearance. Examples are: lye, Chlorox, Draino and ammonia. Acids such as nitric and muriatic used in soldering pastes and in swimming pools are common offenders.

When a child accidently swallows one of these substances, the first mouthful causes intense burning and pain in the throat, making further swallowing almost impossible, but the damage has already been done. Immediate and vigorous treatment is required in the hospital, if more than the inside of the child's mouth is burned. *Do not encourage the child to vomit.* The stomach should not be pumped out as passage of even a soft rubber tube may cause further damage.

It is interesting to note that the alkalies affect mostly the esophagus, while acids affect the stomach. In the acute phase of chemical injuries there are deep ulcerations in the lining of the esophagus and/or stomach, which could in the course of a few weeks or a month produce a stricture in the esophagus. Cortisone is frequently prescribed to reduce the inflammatory reaction and thus the scar tissue. (See Steroids.) However, if narrowing of the esophagus occurs, dilation with a surgical instrument is sometimes necessary.

ACIDOSIS

Acidosis is a blood condition in which the bicarbonate concentration of the blood is below normal. This symptom generally occurs in certain stages of:

1. Diabetes
2. Diarrhea
3. Infections
4. Nephritis
5. Starvation
6. Aspirin poisoning.

The signs and symptoms of acidosis include the following, any one or all of which may be present in various degrees:

1. Rapid breathing which is pauseless in nature—like a dog panting.
2. Drowsiness and restlessness.
3. Fruity odor to the breath—like acetone.
4. Cherry red lips.
5. Dehydration. The signs and symptoms of dehydration include:
   a. Weight loss.
   b. Dryness of the mouth.
   c. Collapsed superficial veins.
   d. Sunken eyes.
   e. Decreased urination.
   f. Diminished skin turgor—loss of normal elasticity.

To determine the extent of acidosis, laboratory studies are correlated with the patient's clinical condition. The underlying illness must be treated as well as the acidosis. Treatment consists of the proper administration of fluids, usually given directly into the patient's vein. In young children it may be difficult for your physician to find a vein in which to inject these fluids. Therefore, once the fluids are started it is necessary that your child be restrained. Do not be frightened when you see this. The restraints are not hurting the child and are only temporary. I am always amazed at how rapidly children respond to fluid therapy.

ADENITIS—MESENTERIC

Mesenteric adenitis is an acute infection of the lymph glands located in the abdomen (belly). These glands are similar to the glands that swell in your neck with certain illnesses. You probably have felt them yourself. Mesenteric adenitis usually occurs in association with an upper respiratory infection. Therefore, it is the commonest cause of abdominal pain in children.

Many times mesenteric adenitis produces the same signs and symptoms as *acute appendicitis:*

1. The pain is at first generalized, often around the navel.
2. The pain may then localize in the right lower part of the abdomen.
3. There may be associated vomiting.
4. Specific changes may occur in the patient's blood count.
5. Fever—101–102 degree range.

Consult a physician whenever abdominal pain is present. Swollen abdominal glands will regress in size in a few days with disappearance of all symptoms. Rest, a light diet, and medication for pain are prescribed. Of course any associated infection is treated.

Because of the similarity of symptoms between mesenteric adenitis and appendicitis, it may be impossible to distinguish between these two conditions. Therefore, a physician may find it necessary to operate, even if he removes a normal appendix. Each doctor will evaluate the situation carefully. A good surgeon will remove approximately fifteen normal appendices in every one hundred operations.

When surgery is performed and a specimen taken, it will auto matically be sent to the pathologist for examination. A pathologist is a medical specialist concerned with studying the nature of disease and the changes in tissues and organs which cause, or are caused by, disease. He examines the tissue by making sections of it and studying it under the microscope.

Surgical exploration does the patient no harm. However, if the diagnosis of appendicitis is missed, the appendix may rupture and cause an infection of the abdominal (belly) cavity called peritonitis. A child with peritonitis is extremely ill and vigorous treatment with antibiotics is necessary to combat the infection. Extended hospital care is necessary.

ADENOIDS

The adenoids are a mass of tissue located in the upper part of the back of the throat. They cannot be seen when the patient opens his mouth and says "ah" unless a mirror is used. The adenoids and tonsils are intimately associated with each other. Adenoiditis means that the adenoids are infected.

The signs and symptoms include fever, sore throat, a foul odor coming from the mouth, and occasionally an associated ear infection. No specific laboratory work is necessary to confirm the diagnosis. Specific treatment consists of antibiotic therapy prescribed by your physician based on whatever organism he feels is causing the infection. The suggestions made under the symptomatic treatment of the common cold are extremely helpful.

The adenoids are frequently enlarged in young children, even when no infection is present. The signs and symptoms are breathing through the mouth and snoring. However, it must be remembered that the young baby is frequently a mouth breather by preference.

Enlarged adenoids block the back of the nose, causing obstruction to the flow of air while breathing. They also press on the eustachian tube which connects the back of the throat with the middle ear. When the eustachian tube is blocked it becomes filled with mucous. Then the normal organisms in the back of the throat migrate via this blocked tube to the middle ear causing recurrent ear infections. This is not a problem in adults because as the child grows older the eustachian tube becomes wider, longer and twisted, making it more difficult for obstruction to occur. A helpful hint that may sometimes shrink the size of the adenoids is the use of high dosages of antihistamine for approximately six weeks. Ask your physician about this.

The adenoids and tonsils, contrary to popular belief, do not exist just to be removed, but serve a useful purpose helping to fight infection. For example, the incidence of rheumatic fever is higher in those children who have had their tonsils and adenoids removed. Since the advent of modern antibiotic therapy, *most children do not need to have their adenoids removed.*

Disease conditions involving the adenoids and/or tonsils become less frequent after five or six years of age. With the passage of time these tissues shrink in size and thus cause less trouble. This, however, must not be used as an excuse to avoid surgery when legitimately indicated.

I have a healthy respect for all surgery, no matter how minor it may be considered, since the child must be put to sleep. It is very easy for bleeding to occur, particularly in the area of the adenoids. Since the adenoids and tonsils are intimately related to each other, the indications for the removal of the adenoids are usually the same as for removal of the tonsils. (See Tonsillitis.)

However, if obstruction to the eustachian tube is present in a child under a few years of age, causing recurring ear infections that do not respond to the usual therapy, including desensitization shots for allergy, the adenoids are often removed and the tonsils left. The reason for this is that a deeper level of anesthesia is necessary for the removal of the tonsils. Thus, by not removing tonsils in the very young child, surgery is made even safer.

Do not expect the removal of the adenoids and/or tonsils to create miracles if there is an underlying disease condition present, such as allergy, unless the allergy is also treated. In the severely allergic child the adenoids and/or tonsils may occasionally grow back.

Some time ago the removal of the adenoids and tonsils was contraindicated in the summer, which was the polio season. Now, the operation may be done any time of the year since epidemics of poliomyelitis are rare and completely preventable.

37

ALLERGIC NOSE—PERENNIAL ALLERGIC RHINITIS (PAR) —HAYFEVER

The mucous membrane which lines the nose becomes swollen and pale when it is affected by allergy. Thus the air passages of the nose become blocked to some degree. When the child cannot get enough air through his nose, he breathes through his mouth, and complains of nasal stuffiness. He may be constantly blowing his nose and using nose drops. A marked watery discharge is usually present. Itching may be intense and constant. When an allergic child rubs his nose he often starts with his hand and continues rubbing until the elbow is reached. This is called an allergic salute. Postnasal drip frequently occurs. This is worse at night and first thing in the morning as the mucous pools in the back of the throat before dripping down. When the child is upright he is more capable of handling this mucous and it seems less severe. The mucous frequently becomes yellow or green, indicating that secondary infestion has occurred. Since the sinuses drain into the nose, they are often involved with secondary infection. This may cause headache of varying degrees over the forehead or over the area below the eyes, corresponding to the position of the frontal and maxillary sinuses.

The diagnosis of nasal allergy is established by correlating a careful history with the typical appearance of the nasal mucous membrane on physical examination. Usually no confirmatory laboratory tests are needed.

When this condition occurs most of the year, it is called perennial allergic rhinitis (PAR). When patients are affected only during certain pollen seasons, the term hayfever is used.

Treatment is aimed at controlling the symptoms. Nose drops are most helpful in relieving the nasal stuffiness. One-quarter per cent of neosynephrine is available in the drugstore without a prescription. In the infant or young child, one drop may be inserted in the nose four times a day. In the older child, two or three drops may be inserted in the nose four times a day. Many other excellent nose drops are available in the drugstore with or without a prescription. Ask your physician about his favorite preparation. Since every child is an individual, one product will occasionally give more relief than another. The excessive use of nose drops, however, may cause a rebound effect. After the initial beneficial effect, the mucous membrane of the nose may become more swollen than before, with worsening of the symptoms.

Antihistamine to control the mucous should be used on a when-necessary basis. Many antihistamines are available in the drugstore without a prescription. A good one is Triaminic. The dosage of Triaminic Syrup is as follows:

1. Under six months of age, an eighth of a teaspoon may be given *four times a day.*
2. A six-month-old baby may be given one-quarter of a teaspoon *four times a day.*
3. Children one to six years of age, one-half teaspoon *every four hours.*
4. Children six to twelve years of age, one teaspoon *every four hours.*

If the same antihistamine is used over a long period of time the child may become resistant to it. If this occurs, change antihistamines. Ask your physician which one he prefers. Antihistamines are not habit-forming and may therefore be used indefinitely. Their only side effect is drowsiness if the dosage is too high.

Occasionally for the immediate relief of acute symptoms steroids (cortisone) may be prescribed by your doctor. However, steroids are not recommended for routine or prolonged use. (See Steroids.)

If secondary infection occurs, antibiotic therapy will be necessary. The choice of antibiotic should be made by the child's physician based upon what organism he feels is causing the infection.

The factors that influence any allergy are listed under Asthma and the Allergic Patient. They should be carefully considered. The practical suggestions discussed under Asthma should also be followed when applicable. Remember there is no cure for an allergic nose, but relief is available. When the condition is severe, causing a constant postnasal drip, chronic lung disease may develop. Therefore, skin testing and desensitization shots are indicated if postnasal drip is persistent in spite of medication, if uncontrollable symptoms make the patient uncomfortable all the time, or if there is associated asthma. (See Asthma and the Allergic Patient.) Nasal allergy is one of the three major symptoms of an allergic patient. Therefore,

39

such a patient has a greater statistical chance of developing the other major symptoms of allergy, namely asthma and eczema, than a non-allergic patient.

ANEMIA—IRON DEFICIENCY

Iron deficiency anemia is completely preventable with sound nutrition. Even though a newborn baby is born with an excessive amount of hemoglobin, his iron stores are very limited. Therefore, by six months of age, the hemoglobin is normally lower. From that point on it is necessary for the baby to receive adequate amounts of iron in the diet to prevent the development of iron deficiency anemia. Unfortunately, there are very few good sources of iron. Milk is totally deficient in iron. Babies who drink more than a quart of milk a day regularly will develop iron deficiency anemia, in spite of the fact that they seem to be chubby and gaining weight. Excellent sources of iron are meat—especially liver—oatmeal, eggs, whole wheat, cabbage and spinach. However, contrary to belief, you would have to eat great quantities of spinach to get an adequate amount of iron. If these foods are rejected, prophylactic iron drops are probably indicated.

The major sign of anemia is pallor. The skin, nail beds and inner aspects of the eyelids are pale. The heart rate may be increased and a heart murmur may develop if the anemia is severe. (See Heart Murmurs.) The heart may also become enlarged because of the extra work it must perform to compensate for the anemia. This is unusual, however, and completely curable. Frequently, anemic children have repeated infections since an adequate level of hemoglobin is necessary to prevent and properly fight infection. WARNING: Do not rule out the possibility of anemia even if the child has a good appetite, normal activity and adequate growth and development.

The diagnosis is established by checking the patient's hemoglobin and examining the red blood cells under the microscope. The serum iron level may also be determined, but this is not necessary in most cases. A child is considered anemic if his hemoglobin is less than ten grams.

Treatment consists of adequate amounts of iron to restore the deficiency and replenish the normal iron stores of the body. Iron

40

is usually given orally, but an injectable form is available. Injectable iron is necessary if the iron given orally is not absorbed properly from the intestinal tract and for the severely anemic child in an effort to avoid blood transfusions. Blood transfusions are only given in emergency situations because they are potentially dangerous. When drops containing iron are given to young babies some darkening of the membrane covering the baby's teeth may occur. This is not serious or permanent. The enamel of the teeth is not affected. Should this darkening or staining occur it may be removed easily. Once a week, place a little baking soda or tooth powder on a small cloth and rub the baby's teeth. The discoloration disappears readily.

There will be a noticeable improvement in the child's appetite as the hemoglobin is restored to a normal level. Of course, the diet must be corrected. There needs to be complete re-education regarding eating habits. If milk has been taken in excessive amounts in preference to solids, it must be drastically reduced. The only way to do this is to suddenly withdraw the usual amount of milk given. Limit the milk to eighteen to twenty-four ounces per day. When drinking milk the baby has just one continuous action: gulp-gulp. When eating solids for the first time the baby must learn how to push the food to the back of his throat before he can swallow. Once solids are eaten well, the amount of milk given may be increased up to one quart per day. Of course an adequate diet must be maintained to prevent recurrence of iron deficiency anemia.

All the changes that may occur with iron deficiency anemia are completely reversible in a short period of time with adequate therapy. No permanent damage occurs.

ANEMIA—SICKLE CELL

In sickle cell anemia abnormally shaped red blood cells are present in the blood, which are easily broken down, causing anemia.

There are periodic crises in which the blood count drops acutely, causing marked pallor. Severe jaundice (yellowness) develops. These crises are accompanied with severe abdominal pain and cramping of the legs. Moderate retardation in physical growth and development is not uncommon.

Sickle cell anemia is hereditary in nature. The red blood cell becomes elongated or sickle-like in appearance at reduced oxygen tension. It occurs predominantly in the Negro race. The diagnosis is confirmed by laboratory studies.

There is no cure for sickle cell anemia. Hospitalization is often necessary during a crisis. A crisis can occur at any time, but fortunately they are infrequent—perhaps a few a year in the average case. A crisis is usually aborted by fluids injected directly into the patient's vein. Blood transfusions are frequently necessary. However, a blood transfusion is not given to maintain an arbitrary level of hemoglobin. It is only given to allow the child to function adequately in his environment. Children with sickle cell anemia will adapt to a much lower level of hemoglobin than normal children are accustomed to. They will adjust their activities to compensate for this.

Infections are more common because of the anemia. They are treated vigorously with antibiotics. With good care and no complications, a normal life span is to be expected.

Sickle cell anemia should not be confused with the sickle cell trait. The sickle cell trait is the tendency of an individual's red blood cells to assume the sickle form under conditions of reduced oxygen tension. It also is hereditary in nature and occurs predominantly in the Negro race. However, no anemia is present. Individuals with the sickle cell trait are symptom-free and require no treatment.

ANTIBIOTIC THERAPY—PRINCIPLES OF

Antibiotics do not represent a magic or rapid cure-all for all infectious diseases. They are of no value in viral infections such as the common cold. Antibiotics are indicated in bacterial infections. The antibiotic chosen is determined by the organisms causing the infection based upon your physician's judgment. If he is in doubt as to the exact cause of an infection, or if the patient is seriously ill, cultures will be obtained. A culture is a means of growing the bacteria in the laboratory so that it may be identified. The bacteria's sensitivity to different antibiotics is then determined in the test tube. In most cases, however, antibiotic therapy is started prior to obtaining the laboratory results. Necessary adjustments are made later on by correlating the patient's clinical response with the test results.

Some antibiotics such as penicillin are bacteriacidal. They

actually kill the bacteria. Other antibiotics such as terramycin are bacteriostatic. They inhibit the growth of the bacteria, but do not actually kill them.

The dosage of antibiotics is calculated according to the patient's weight. WARNING: Do not exceed the dose prescribed by your physican. The idea that if the prescribed amount is good, more is better, may lead to serious or life-threatening side effects. Most antibiotics are given every six hours to maintain a therapeutic blood level as time is required for absorption to take place from the gastro-intestinal tract. If antibiotics are only given during the waking hours —by that I mean four times a day—a therapeutic level is often not maintained because of the elapsed time between the last dose at night and the absorption of the antibiotic into the blood stream in the morning. This may allow the bacteria causing the infection to become resistant to the specific antibiotic. A few oral antibiotics have been developed which may be given every twelve hours, or once a day.

Most antibiotics may be given with other medications. If there should be interference with a particular antibiotic's mode of action, your physician will tell you to give that medication separately. Most antibiotics can also be given before, with, or after meals. In un-usual cases your physician will instruct you.

One of the most important principles of antibiotic therapy is its duration. A minimum of five days of treatment is usually required. If therapy is stopped after two or three days without your physician's permission because the patient seems well, relapses or complications frequently occur requiring additional antibiotics. This type of in-termittent treatment promotes resistance to the antibiotic and may contribute to drug allergies in the patient.

Most doctors realize that antibiotics are expensive. Therefore, they will prescribe just enough medicine to last the appropriate amount of time. This means that the physician wants the patient to finish all the medicine he prescribes unless he instructs the patient to consult him in a few days after taking part of it. If your physician asks you—the parent—to call and give him a progress report, do not fail to do this because the child feels better. Your physician wants to know that the medication is working properly. He may want to give you further instructions.

The problem of an allergic reaction to an antibiotic is far outweighed by its usefulness. There is no perfect medicine. Allergies to antibiotics are acquired and not inherited. Therefore, if the parents are allergic to penicillin, it does not mean that their child will be. Clarify this thought in your own mind to avoid unnecessary fear. In addition, an allergic reaction the first time a medicine is prescribed is rare.

I want to allay the average person's unfounded fear of penicillin. Penicillin allergy is not a significant problem in children; the incidence is put at one in one hundred thousand. This is even less a problem than I believed prior to research of the literature. Allergic reactions to any drugs may be manifested by any of the following symptoms:

1. Giant hives or welts with associated itching.
2. Vomiting.
3. Cramping.
4. Swelling around the lips or mouth.
5. Interference with normal breathing and heart action in severe cases.

If a suspected allergic reaction to antibiotics occurs, stop the medicine. Inform your physician immediately. Allergic reactions can be immediately counteracted by injectable adrenalin and/or cortisone. Antihistamines are also prescribed. Besides these potent classes of drugs to combat any allergy, there is a specific enzyme which counteracts penicillin called penicillinase. This product is sold as Neutrapen. It is intended for the control and treatment of allergic reactions to penicillin. With these drugs we have enough weapons to satisfactorily combat any allergic reaction to penicillin or other drugs. If an allergic reaction occurs the same antibiotic will not be prescribed again. Therapy, however, can be safely continued with other medication.

I personally feel that all patients with suspected allergy to antibiotics should be examined by the doctor. Many cases diagnosed over the phone turn out to be something else. In children it is foolish to assume that any rash is due to an allergic reaction when the rash may well represent some childhood illness. There is no reason why the physician should reduce his armamentarium for the treatment of infectious diseases unnecessarily.

Certain antibiotics have a tendency to cause loose stools. This is because the antibiotics, besides killing the harmful bacteria which cause infection, also kill the normal bacteria which must be present in our intestinal tract if we are to have normal bowel movements. Take all of the antibiotic, however, unless the diarrhea is severe. If necessary, Kaopectate and paregoric may be given either separately or together. The stools will return to normal a few days after the antibiotic is completed. Remember that excessive fruit juice also causes loose stools. If this occurs, carbonated beverages make fine substitutes.

The bacteria which causes infections are divided into two categories, gram positive and gram negative, depending upon what color stain they absorb in the laboratory. Those antibiotics which are primarily effective against only gram positive organisms, such as penicillin, are not considered broad spectrum antibiotics because they do not have a wide range of activity. A broad spectrum antibiotic is effective against both gram positive and gram negative bacteria.

Parents should not be afraid of giving antibiotics wondering what will happen if a more serious infection occurs. Many bacteria which have been resistant to previous antibiotic therapy are susceptible to newer drugs that are being marketed yearly. In addition, the dosage of a particular antibiotic can usually be pushed to higher levels in stubborn cases. A list of current popular antibiotics available commercially includes: Bacitracin, Chloromycetin, Colistin, Erythromycin, Furadantin, Ilosone, Kanamycin, Keflin, Lincocin, Loridine, Neomycin, Novobiocin, Humatin, at least ten different kinds of penicillin, Polymyxin, Ristocetin, Streptomycin, Sulfa, Tetracyclines, various modifications of Tetracycline and Vancomycin.

Most physicians will not prescribe antibiotics over the telephone. Your physician is a skilled clinician and in most cases must see the child to decide if antibiotic therapy is necessary and, if so, what antibiotic is the drug of choice. It is usually impossible for a physician to make such an important decision over the telephone. The same principle applies to renewal of a prescription some time later. It is amazing how often I have telephone calls from a parent asking me to renew a prescription for an antibiotic because the child has the same illness again. The symptoms may be the same but the cause (etiology) may be different, thus requiring another antibiotic. I refuse all such requests. Most parents accept this reasoning and realize that this principle is in the best interest of their child.

Certain antibiotics occasionally have adverse side effects. Your physician does not prescribe such antibiotics indiscriminately, but they are sometimes necessary when a patient has failed to respond to the usual therapy, and in the more serious infections such as meningitis. If the parents are concerned about the action of any particular antibiotic they should discuss it with their physician. The medication should not be stopped arbitrarily by the parent because of fear based on rumor.

If your child is on antibiotics for a prolonged period of time your physician will probably recommend that his blood and urine be checked at regular intervals.

APPENDICITIS

Appendicitis means inflammation (infection) of the appendix. The appendix is a worm-like projection from the large bowel. Acute appendicitis is the most common surgical condition in children. It is rare under one year of age and it is more common in the male child. The disease is characterized by a sudden onset of generalized abdominal pain which is often located around the navel. Later the pain becomes localized in the right lower part of the abdomen (belly). Frequently the pain is accompanied by nausea and vomiting. The temperature is usually between 101 and 102 degrees.

On physical examination rebound tenderness is found in the right lower part of the abdomen. When your physician presses on the belly wall and suddenly lets go, it hurts. A significant degree of muscle spasm is present. On rectal examination point tenderness may be found. The white blood cell count which shows how the body is fighting infection may be elevated. Any change in this test is significant. In suspected cases, this blood test may be repeated at frequent intervals. Silent pneumonia may cause belly pain. The pain is not felt in the chest, but is referred to the abdomen (belly) by a group of nerves. Therefore, it is advisable that young children in whom the diagnosis of appendicitis is suspected have an X ray of the chest.

All suspected cases of appendicitis should be hospitalized for observation. Time is required for the clinical picture to unfold. The diet will be restricted to clear liquids as long as the possibility of surgery exists. The only acceptable treatment is removal of the appendix. This is called an appendectomy.

The outlook for complete and early recovery in infants and children is excellent. Hospitalization will usually not exceed five to seven days.

The diagnosis of acute appendicitis is very difficult. The lymph glands in the abdomen may swell with any upper respiratory infection causing abdominal pain. This is called mesenteric adenitis. Sometimes it is impossible to distinguish between these two conditions. Therefore, a good surgeon may remove normal appendices. (See Adenitis, Mesenteric.) The risk of surgery is far less than the possible risk and complications of a ruptured appendix. A ruptured appendix causes peritonitis which is an infection of the abdominal (belly) cavity. This is a serious illness. Vigorous treatment with antibiotics is necessary.

ARTHRITIS—RHEUMATOID

Arthritis means inflammation of the joints. Rheumatoid arthritis is a rare disease in children. It is more common in females than males.

The onset may be acute with fluctuating fever and typically red swollen joints, or insidious with slow indolent involvement of single or multiple joints without fever. The joints most often involved are the knees, fingers and feet. In some cases there is a typical flat red rash that suddenly appears with the occurrence of fever, and rapidly subsides as the fever disappears. The individual lesions are transitory, even if the rash persists for weeks or months. As the disease progresses there may be involvement of all the joints and marked dimunition in the size of the muscles from lack of use, with resulting deformity. The disease is characterized by remissions and exacerbations. Fortunately, many months may go by without symptoms. The exact cause of arthritis is unknown, although constitutional susceptibility, infection, injury and allergy have been suspected of playing roles. A typical X-ray appearance of the joints may be demonstrated as the disease progresses. There is no specific laboratory test that will confirm the diagnosis. The sedimentation rate, which is a nonspecific blood test of activity, is an excellent

47

way of following the disease process. The disease is active when the sedimentation rate is elevated.

There is no cure for rheumatoid arthritis. The therapy of this disease can be divided into four parts—rest, physiotherapy, emotional support, and drug therapy. The amount of rest needed depends upon the individual child. A child acutely ill with multiple joint involvement and fever should have complete bed rest. A child with involvement of only one or two joints without fever may do well with additional sleep at night or a nap during the day. Rest is indicated even though weight bearing joints such as the hips are not involved. When rest is no longer necessary, there should be gradual resumption of activity.

A difficult concept for parents to understand is that the additional rest must also be accompanied by proper exercise. Passive exercise, i.e., the moving of the joint by another person, may be all that will be tolerated early in the treatment. It is important to try to maintain a full range of motion of each joint through proper exercise. Some joint pain after exercise should be anticipated. If this pain does not last over an hour, there is nothing to worry about. Heat is valuable in decreasing stiffness before exercise. A hot tub bath may be used at home, or hot towels may be applied to individual joints for fifteen or twenty minutes.

As in any chronic disease, emotional support of the child is necessary. The parents should discuss their feelings with a physician particularly interested in dealing with attitudes—a clinical psychologist or psychiatrist. The parents must learn how to control their own anxiety or the child will become anxious too. Maintain proper communication with your child and discuss the disease process openly. It is better to get fears out in the open than keep them bottled up within.

Aspirin is still the drug of choice for control of fever and pain. If aspirin is irritating to the stomach, many excellent substitutes are available. Cortisone has been referred to as the rich man's aspirin. This is not really so because cortisone is a much more potent drug than aspirin and can thus prevent crippling in many patients. However, contrary to popular belief, cortisone does not cure arthritis; it alleviates the symptoms. (See Steroids.) Some drugs which are used to fight malaria have also proved to be of value in the treatment of rheumatoid arthritis.

Depending upon the clinical course, arthritis may or may not be a crippling disease. With proper care many deformities can be avoided and the child can lead a useful life. It is important that a consistent long-term approach be used. The child should see a physician at regular intervals so that all the advances of modern medicine can be used to help him.

ARTIFICIAL RESPIRATION AND EXTERNAL CARDIAC MASSAGE

A patient who is making any spontaneous respiratory effort should not receive artificial respiration. The fundamentals of artificial respiration are:

1. Make sure that the airway is clear.
2. Provide proper ventilation.

Before starting artificial respiration in a patient who is not breathing make sure that there is no material in his throat that is obstructing the airway. Hold the patient's head down, opening his mouth. Run your finger over his tongue to remove any foreign material. If a metal or plastic airway is available, it is then inserted. Resuscitation is then carried out with the patient lying down with his head low.

The quickest way to give artificial respiration is with mouth to mouth breathing. Extend the patient's head backward, hold the jaw forward and blow air into his mouth with enough force to expand the chest. Distention of the patient's stomach may be prevented by gentle pressure on the upper left side of the belly after each breath.

In a severely depressed patient, external cardiac massage is carried out at the same time. Kneel beside the patient, place one hand over the lower third of the breast bone. Place the heel of your other hand on top of your first hand. Now press downward using the weight of your body to depress the breast bone one to one and one-half inches. This action compresses the heart between the breast bone and the back bone. This forces the blood out of the heart into the lungs. Now release the pressure lifting your hands slightly. This allows the patient's chest to expand fully, and the heart to refill with blood. Repeat the cycle about sixty to eighty times a minute. If you are the only person present, you should rapidly ventilate the patient's lungs by mouth to mouth resuscitation followed by external cardiac massage for about a minute. Then stop the external cardiac massage and ventilate the patient again. Continue to alternate these life saving measures. There is no need to synchronize these measures unless someone else is present.

The above emergency first aid should be carried on if necessary until trained medical help is available. Do not give up. A patient may start spontaneous respiration even an hour or two later.

ASPIRIN

Approximately twenty-one tons of aspirin are used daily in the United States. The public probably fails to consider aspirin a drug. Fortunately, aspirin is probably the safest drug there is. Most physicians, if they were to be isolated on an island and could only have available to them one drug, would choose aspirin.

Aspirin, in addition to controlling fever and pain, has an anti-inflammatory effect. Aspirin is a useful drug in most illnesses of children. For example, it may be used for control of fever and pain in chicken pox, mumps, German measles, measles, whooping cough, diphtheria, tonsillitis, pharangitis, adenoiditis, pneumonia, cystitis, infectious mononeucleosis, tuberculosis, scarlet fever, meningitis, typhoid fever, etc. It is also used for its specific anti-inflammatory effect in rheumatic fever and rheumatoid arthritis.

The cost of aspirin varies a great deal. Buy the cheapest brand. No aspirin tablet is more potent than another. The proper dosage of aspirin for a child one to five years of age, providing he is of normal weight for his age, is one baby aspirin per year of age until age five. The dosage is repeated every four hours as needed. After age five one adult aspirin may be given every four hours. For a child less than a year of age, it is important not to give too much aspirin. For a six-month-old child I recommend one-half of a baby aspirin every four to six hours. For a child less than six months of age, I recommend one-quarter of a baby aspirin every four to six hours. To make the administration of aspirin tablets easier, one aspirin may be dissolved in a tablespoon of water. To give one-quarter of an aspirin give one teaspoon of this solution. Be sure, however, the aspirin is thoroughly mixed with the water. For younger children the administration of aspirin may be made easier if the aspirin is mixed with applesauce, honey or jam. Aspirin may also be absorbed from the rectum if too much stool is not present. This is the preferred route of administration if the child has been vomiting, since aspirin may occasionally irritate the stomach. Rectal suppositories are available in the drugstore without a prescription. One five-grain suppository equals four baby aspirins. Double the usual dosage may be given rectally. Contrary to popular belief, aspirin is not available as a liquid because it is unstable. Chemically, aspirin is acetyl-salicylic acid. So-called "liquid aspirin" is another type of drug that helps control fever. I do not recommend it as it is not as effective as aspirin, tempra or tylenol. Baby Bufferin in the same dosages may be substituted for baby aspirin.

ASPIRIN POISONING

Accidents are the leading cause of death in children. The accidental ingestion of aspirin is the commonest accident. Your physician should be called immediately. Try to establish how much aspirin has been taken. Determine roughly how many tablets were in the bottle and how many are left. From this information your physician will calculate the approximate amount taken and relate it to the child's weight. If your doctor decides an overdose of aspirin is a possibility, immediate treatment is started.

If the accidental ingestion of aspirin is discovered before the stomach is completely empty, it should be emptied to prevent further absorption of the drug. Vomiting may be induced by giving ipecac. I believe everyone should have a poison control kit at home which contains ipecac and charcoal. An ipechar Poison Control Kit is commercially available in your drugstore. (See Poisoning.) Your doctor may prefer, depending on the circumstances, to wash out the patient's stomach by passing a soft tube through his mouth or nose into the stomach. He then washes the stomach out until all the accidentally ingested material is removed. This procedure is not dangerous and will not hurt your child.

The level of aspirin in the patient's blood may be determined when indicated. This is called the salicylate level. If it should be high, the child should be admitted to the hospital for observation.

The signs of aspirin poisoning do not occur immediately, but are insidious in onset. Shallow, rapid respirations similar to a dog panting occurs which denotes changes in the body's acid-base balance. This is usually treated by injecting fluids directly into the patient's vein. (See Acidosis.) If symptoms related to the central nervous system, such as high fever, coma and convulsions develop, it is sometimes necessary to perform an exchange transfusion or employ an artificial kidney to lower the salicylate level of the blood.

Once the patient has recovered, relapses are impossible unless an additional toxic dose of aspirin is ingested. Unfortunately, I have treated the same child more than once for aspirin poisoning.

ASTHMA AND THE ALLERGIC PATIENT

Surveys indicate that over 3,000,000 people suffer from bronchial asthma in the United States. The majority of these patients develop their disease in childhood.

In asthma, excessive mucous is produced in the chest—enough to form a mucous plug. When the patient breathes in (inhales air) the bronchioles elongate allowing air to pass by the mucous. When the patient blows air out of the lungs (exhales) the bronchioles shorten and close down on the mucous plug. A ball valve type of obstruction is thereby created causing the wheeze. The patient has difficulty in getting air out. If the parent places his hand on the child's chest, he will often be able to feel the mucous.

All that wheezes is not asthma; other conditions such as a foreign body caught in the airway, tumors and cystic fibrosis need to be considered. (See Cystic Fibrosis.) Asthma should also be differentiated from asthmatic bronchitis. Some people call this asthma, but wheezing is only present when there is an associated respiratory infection. This is particularly common during the first three years of life. The wheezing will stop when the infection is properly treated. (See Asthmatic Bronchitis.)

The onset of asthma may be gradual or sudden. Asthma may occur in children who have never exhibited allergic symptoms before. The frequency of attacks will vary depending on age, cause, associated infection, and duration of the disease.

Attacks may occur seasonally with an increase in the pollen count from specific plants, or throughout the year. It is harder to control those children who have attacks of asthma seasonally. Attacks of asthma may be infrequent even if the exposure to the offending allergic pollen is continuous. Food allergies can also cause asthma and are especially important in children under one year of age. In considering allergies to food I like to think of an intolerance to a particular food. A child intolerant to some foods one month may not be two or three months later. It should be noted that 50 per cent of all allergic children will develop wheezing sometime in their lives and that children who had eczema early in life or an allergic nose tend to have more severe cases of asthma.

The incidence of allergy in children is high. However, children have a very good response to adequate management. Four out of five children treated with allergy injections are free of asthma by adolescence. Many people believe that children will outgrow allergies. It is true that at puberty, because of the hormones produced, there may be some changes in the course of allergies, but this is really not outgrowing them. Children may outgrow specific allergies, but other allergies are apt to take their place. It is best to consider that once a patient is allergic, he is always allergic. Hay fever adds to the persistence of asthma. Eczema has no bearing on the outcome of asthma. I believe that in 95 per cent or more of the cases, chronic lung disease can be prevented with proper control of infection, desensitization to specific allergies and consideration of the emotional aspects of the disease.

I like to explain allergies as various steps going up the mountain, with each step representing specific allergies. If the child is on the first or the tenth step, there may be no signs and symptoms. An additional step, however, will cause clinical signs and symptoms. Naturally, the number of steps required varies with each individual. In controlling the allergic child, the physician helps him descend the steps of the mountain, thereby eliminating the clinical signs and symptoms, but does not cure him. However, elimination of the clinical signs and symptoms should prevent chronic lung disease.

Influencing Factors

Allergic, mechanical, infectious, and emotional factors are involved in cases of allergies. All must be considered in the care of the whole child. A list of factors include:

1. Inhalants which are breathed in and irritate the respiratory system. Pollens, molds, house dust, and animal epidermals are most important.

2. Ingestants—Food and other products digested in the stomach. The ten common food offenders, in order, are: milk, chocolate, cola, corn, egg, citrus, legumes (pea, peanut), tomato, wheat, cinnamon and artificial food color. Some medications at times may possibly be important.

3. Infection—Acute. Chronic infection is seldom a problem.

4. Congenital abnormalities which may interfere with normal respirations; for example, a pigeon chest.

5. Over exertion.

6. Metabolic factors such as occur in cystic fibrosis and low levels of gamma globulin. (See Cystic Fibrosis and Hypogammaglobulinemia.)

7. Irritants such as soap, tobacco smoke, adhesive tape, jewelry, and strong odors such as paint.

8. Environmental changes in the humidity and temperature.

9. Hereditary or constitutional factors. Children do not inherit allergies, but there is usually a family history of allergic problems. If one child in the family is allergic, the other children will probably be allergic sometime in their lives.

10. Psychological factors. In any chronic illness feelings develop about possible restrictions or the frequent use of medication. The child has a right to be afraid when he is struggling for enough oxygen.

Evaluation of the Allergic Patient

A complete history and physical examination must be done. The history will elucidate such things as when the attacks occur, the frequency, the duration, the amount of respiratory distress, response to treatment, family background, recurrent infections and diet. Variations from the normal range of height and weight will be noted as well as the general appearance of the patient. Some laboratory studies which are of value, but not indicated in every patient are:

1. *A complete blood count (CBC).* This will give information regarding the white cells and hemoglobin. It will help the physician distinguish between a child who is chronically ill, anemic, and

allergic. There is a marked increase in a specific type of white blood cell called an eosinophile in an allergic child.

2. *Sedimentation rate.* This is a nonspecific blood test of disease activity.

3. *Urinalysis.* Abnormal cells may appear in the urine of allergic children.

4. *Nose and throat cultures.* It is important to determine if there are any abnormal bacteria in the back of the throat which are causing repeated attacks of infection.

5. *Nasal smear for eosinophiles.* There is often an increase in the eosinophiles in the mucous of the nose. (See Number 1.)

6. *Sweat test.* This is a test that is diagnostic for cystic fibrosis which can mimic asthma. (See Cystic Fibrosis of the Pancreas.)

7. *Electrophoretic pattern for gamma globulin.* This test performed on the blood measures the ability of the body to manufacture antibodies for protection against disease. It may be low in allergic children. (See Hypogammaglobulinemia.)

8. *Studies of pulmonary function.* This will determine the lung capacity. Is the lung capacity decreased due to chronic lung disease?

9. *Stool examination.* There is often an increase in the eosinophiles in the stools of an allergic child. (See Number 1 above.)

10. *X rays of the chest.* In my opinion every allergic child should have an X ray of the chest. It should be repeated on a routine basis, approximately once a year, depending upon the patient's clinical condition. Comparison of films is extremely important in evaluating the disease process.

11. *X ray of the sinuses:* To rule out any masses that may lead to obstruction of the sinuses.

12. *Tuberculin test:* (See Tuberculosis.)

13. *Skin tests:* One method of skin testing employs a small scratch on the patient's back. The outer layer of skin is just barely broken, without drawing blood. The material to be tested for is then dropped on the scratch. Thirty minutes later any reaction that occurs is interpreted and compared to a control. The reactions are graded on a zero to four plus basis. Zero means no reaction, four plus means a marked reaction. I prefer this technique because if the child has a severe allergic reaction to any extract it may be wiped off. Another technique consists of injecting an extract of the material to be tested for between the layers of skin. The reactions are interpreted the same way. The specific tests performed by each

55

physician will depend upon those pollens that are common where you live. For example, in Florida there is more emphasis placed on skin tests for molds than need be in New York City. The average physician probably tests for about seventy-five possible offenders. The commonest offenders in children are: house dust, ragweed, the normal bacteria in the back of one's throat, dog hair, cat hair, and fungi in the warm, humid climates.

Skin testing for foods is particularly important in children under a year of age. They are almost always done by the scratch method. I have some theoretical objections to skin testing for foods. The products of digestion are different from the extracts that may be prepared. However, many physicians have good results.

In most physician's offices the skin tests are performed by trained assistants. The physician will usually interpret the reactions himself. An extract is then prepared for each patient based on the results of the tests. These extracts may take a number of weeks to prepare so do not try to rush the doctor.

Practical Suggestions. Ask your physician which suggestions must be followed and which are worth a try at some time or other, depending on your child's clinical condition. It is impossible to rank these suggestions in any order of importance:

1. All toys should be hypoallergenic. Stuffed toys should be avoided.

2. All new furniture cushions throughout the house should be made of foam rubber. The child's mattress should be of foam rubber or incased in plastic. Plastic cases are available in most department stores.

3. Clothing and other materials should not be stored in the allergic child's room.

4. Place a heating rod in the closets to control fungi. It costs only pennies a day.

5. Create a dust-free room. Ideally, this type of room would have a metal bed and a wooden chair. This may be extreme, but certainly the floor should be bare, or only have cotton rugs that can be washed once a week. If there are curtains on the windows, they should also be washed once a week.

6. Use a special spray such as Dust Seal to help control house dust. (L.S. Green Associates, 160 W. 57th Street, New York, N.Y. 10019.)

7. Clean the house when the patient is outside.

8. Keep the child inside on extremely windy days when the pollen count is bound to be high.

9. Antihistamines should be immediately employed at the first sign of a cold, running nose or sneezing, as directed by your physician.

10. Take the child to his physician at the first sign of illness to control any associated infection early.

11. Eliminate shell fish, chocolate, nuts and peanut butter from the diet even if skin testing for foods has not been done.

12. Try an elimination diet. Omit one group of foods at a time for a week to see if there is any improvement. This is a diagnostic tool as well as a method of treatment.

13. Consider the emotional aspects of asthma. Some psychiatrists have stated that wheezing represents the suppressed cry of the child for mother's help. This does not mean that all allergic children have serious emotional problems—but some do. Certainly in any chronic disease feelings and attitudes will develop about the illness that should be dealt with. No child should be permitted to use prolonged illness for personal gain and gratification. For example, if a child's request is denied he may be able to precipitate an attack of asthma that frightens the parents into granting his desires. If this occurs, professional help is needed from a clinical psychologist or child psychiatrist. (See Psychological Testing.)

14. Moving from state to state because of allergies is rarely recommended. It is true that when the environment is changed the patient may improve for a couple of months because he has moved away from some of his offending allergies. However, he will usually become sensitized to different allergies in his new environment in short order. Sometimes living in different parts of the same community may be helpful. For example, in Fort Lauderdale, Florida, the allergic child does best near the ocean where the air is relatively pollen-free, as compared to the western part of town near the Everglades, from which many pollens come that have not been identified. If attacks of allergies are always precipitated by a change in temperature and humidity, and uncontrollable with desensitization injections, moving may be considered. This idea, however, needs to be discussed with an expert.

15. No dogs or cats are to be kept inside or outside the house. *This is a cardinal principle of allergy control*, even if the skin tests for dog and cat hair show no sensitivity. Many parents and children have developed an attachment to a loved dog or cat, but the psychological manifestations that may occur due to the loss of such

a pet are far outweighed by the advantages of giving the dog or cat to another family who does not have an allergic child. There is a popular old wives' tale that patients quote all the time—that a Chihuahua dog helps relieve wheezing. This is utter nonsense. Pets should be limited to fish and turtles. Avoid all furry animals.

16. Chores should be assigned taking into consideration the patient's allergic history. If the patient is allergic to grass he should not mow the lawn.

17. Overwhelming exposure to the offending agents should be prohibited. A child severely allergic to weeds probably should not go hiking or camping.

18. The child should avoid other children with colds as much as possible. In the allergic patient the mucous membrane of the entire respiratory tree is going to be slightly swollen and red at times, making the patient more susceptible to infection. Avoid excessive chilling.

19. Obtain a yearly immunization against the flu virus.

20. Avoid using sprays such as Gulf Spray, Flit and aerosol bombs because of the pyrethrum in them.

21. Use non-allergic cosmetics such as Almay, Marcelle or An Ex, which can be purchased at most drugstores if any sensitivity to orris root is present.

22. Air condition your house. A letter from your physician will establish this as a necessary medical expense on your tax return. Leave the air conditioning on even if the child becomes sick. Do not be concerned about chilling in going from an air conditioned place to one that is not.

Treatment—Acute Attack

The treatment of asthma depends upon the severity of the symptoms. There are three main classes of drugs:

1. Adrenalin and like compounds.
2. The bronchodilators.
3. Steroids (Cortisone).

The first task of the physician is to control the acute attack. To do this early recognition and treatment of asthma at its onset is most important. Parents must learn to recognize the impending signs so that it may be aborted with simple treatment. If the attack becomes severe, the milder methods of treatment are usually not effective.

An injection of adrenalin is the drug of choice for all acute attacks. It should be given under the supervision of a physician and not by the parents at home. The dosage of adrenalin is determined by the weight of the patient. It may be repeated fifteen minutes later if necessary. If no improvement has occurred by that time, further injections of adrenalin will probably be of no value.

When the patient receives adrenalin he should be told that he will feel his heart pound, since adrenalin increases the heart rate. In addition the child will look pale around the lips because adrenalin constricts the blood vessels. Adrenalin, also known as epinephrine, is so specific for asthma that it is considered a diagnostic test. In other words, if adrenalin relieves the wheezing the diagnosis is asthma.

The main advantage of adrenalin is that it acts rapidly. Relief is usually obtained in a few minutes. Unfortunately, its duration of action is short, a matter of hours. However, oral medicines chemically related to adrenalin are available. They are extremely popular and often prescribed after some of the initial wheezing is relieved.

Ephedrine is similar in its action to adrenalin except it is too slow acting for the treatment of acute attacks. The action of ephedrine is more prolonged. Ephedrine often stimulates the patient. Therefore, it is usually mixed in equal parts with some type of sedation such as phenobarbital.

Theophylline and aminophylline are bronchodilators that are effective in the treatment of acute attacks. The advantages of these drugs are that they may be given directly into the patient's vein, orally, or by rectal suppository. However, the dosage must be carefully regulated to prevent intoxication with these drugs. The symptoms of overdosage include:

1. Fever.
2. Restlessness.
3. Vomiting of coffee ground type material.
4. Dehydration.
5. Convulsions.
6. Coma.

Cortisone (steroids) is the most potent weapon physicians have in their armamentarium for the treatment of asthma and related allergies. Fortunately, allergic patients who really need steroids tolerate them well. However, steroids are not used indiscriminately because there are many side effects with prolonged use. (See Steroids.) This should not, however, make parents afraid of the occasional use of steroids, orally or by injection. Certainly, cortisone for a few days is not going to cause any trouble. It is going to do the patient a world of good when medically indicated as determined by your physician's judgment. Cortisone has the reputation of being a miracle drug, and it is. However, cortisone does not cure asthma—it helps control it.

Expectorants that help the patient bring up the thick mucous secretions are most helpful. A child should be encouraged to take fluids by mouth, both for their expectorant action and to prevent dehydration. Milk should not be given because it produces mucous.

Antihistamines, which are drugs used to help dry up mucous, are not effective in the treatment of acute attacks, and may be harmful due to their drying action. However, antihistamines have a very important place in the prevention of attacks.

Infection is almost always present in children with acute asthma. Antibiotic is usually prescribed. (See Antibiotics.) Sedation may be desirable to allay anxiety. The tranquilizers are excellent on a short-term basis, but are no substitute for dealing with the underlying feelings on a long-term basis.

Intermittent positive pressure breathing (IPPB), also known as inhalation therapy, is a very valuable adjunct to the treatment of asthma. I like to describe this as a mechanical cleaning out of the mucous plugs in the lung. A machine is triggered each time the patient inhales, which causes air or oxygen under increased pressure, along with any medication that may be prescribed in mist form to be delivered directly to the lungs. The amount of the pressure is adjusted by the therapist. Treatments may be given as often as necessary. IPPB therapy allows for improved air exchange, more uniform aeration of the lungs and increased bronchial drainage. This type of machine is not recommended for home use as it is possible to damage the lung if too much pressure is used.

Most physicians are against the use of nebulizer aerosol devices. I use no nebulizer and attempt to stop their use in all patients. This is the type of medication which is administered by a Freon powered pressured aerosol device which delivers a given dosage of medication for inhalation. Children often use nebulization excessively by themselves and become too dependent upon it.

Postural drainage often works wonders in clearing mucous from the lungs. To accomplish this the head must be considerably lower than the chest. A simple way of doing this is to place the child over a half dozen pillows with his head remaining on the bed. The child stays in this position as long as mucous is being caught, usually about fifteen minutes.

The most frequently forgotten ingredient in the care of asthma today is rest. Parents should not expect the above medications or treatments to work miracles without the cooperation of the patient. This means rest in bed when the child is sick. A sick child should not be outside playing or running around the house. However, bathroom privileges and meals at the table are fine in most cases.

If your house has an air conditioner use it, weather permitting. If not, a vaporizer may be of value. (See Colds—treatment, for a detailed discussion of vaporizers.) A window air conditioner and vaporizer is not effective when used simultaneously. The air conditioner's filter must be changed once a month or more, or a washable filter used that is cleaned as frequently. It is amazing, no matter how immaculate a housekeeper you may be, the dust and pollen that is collected.

I believe that most children with asthma under one year of age should be hospitalized for safety's sake. The little guy does not have the same ability to fight infection, fight for air and maintain adequate hydration as the older child. Hospitalization for the older child is indicated if there is respiratory distress, or if your physician deems it advisable for any other reason. The signs and symptoms of respiratory distress are a sucking in, in the neck, between the ribs and under the rib cage and moving in and out of the nose as the child breathes. Under these circumstances, additional oxygen is necessary. It is obviously too risky to set up an oxygen tent in the home.

Treatment for Chronic Asthma

The treatment of chronic asthma consists of treating the attacks as described above, which occur frequently, and organizing a plan for the prevention of chronic lung disease. Your physician must be consulted at the first sign of trouble. Medication must always be available in the home and accompany the child on any trips.

Sometimes a child with chronic asthma will respond well to prophylactic antibiotic therapy. Chest infection is sometimes prevented this way. If attacks are frequent and severe, maintenance dosage of cortisone (steroid) may be necessary. This certainly is a must if the child is developing chronic lung disease. Once chronic changes have occurred in the lungs, they are not reversible. However, additional changes may be prevented.

Skin testing and hypodesensitization shots are mandatory in an effort to prevent chronic lung disease. (See Hypodesensitization Therapy.) It is also important to deal with the child's feelings and to teach him how to live with a chronic illness. (See Evaluation of the Allergic Patient #12.) Breathing exercises are important. (See Breathing Exercises.)

I do not believe in restricting athletics or physical activity in the allergic child if at all possible. If it is obvious that with over exertion an attack of asthma occurs, the child can be taught to avoid this. Swim training has been studied in the severely asthmatic child. It has been proven that there are no adverse effects. In fact, it may have a number of beneficial side effects, including improvement in sleep, appetite, and behavior.

Complacency on the part of the parents may occur in chronic asthma. Although the parents are accustomed to the child wheezing, it must not be ignored. Wishful thinking and denial will not prevent chronic lung disease. For a specific discussion of chronic lung disease see Bronchiectasis and Emphysema.

It is important that a long-term approach be used. The child should see a physician at regular intervals so that all the advances of modern medicine can be used to help him.

If, in spite of all these measures, adequate results are not obtained, hospitalization in a special institution for asthmatics should be considered. There are a number of such hospitals, particularly in Denver, Colorado. There may be one near you. Ask your physician. The parents must realize that if such a recommendation is necessary, all approaches to prevent recurrent asthma have failed. Therefore, if the child is to lead a normal and fruitful life, separation from the family members must be tolerated by all concerned. I have sent a number of patients to these special hospitals. They have all returned home considerably improved. Do not let your own anxiety prevent proper treatment. Talk over any possible feelings of guilt with a clinical psychologist or psychiatrist. Do not become sucked in by unethical clinics or quacks that promise cures or use machines with flashing lights and noise makers. The chances are that any person who promises a cure is a quack. If in doubt contact your local medical society. These quacks are now frequently locating themselves outside the United States, along the Texas border.

Hypodesensitization Therapy

No person in this world has a cure for allergies. Allergies, however, can be controlled well enough in the vast majority of cases to prevent chronic lung disease. It must be remembered that the goals of the physician may be more long-ranged than the goals of the parents. The parents want to eliminate the attacks of asthma, and the physician does too, but he is probably more practical in his approach. He must think of the child's future and the prevention of additional problems.

In hypodesensitization therapy an extract is made for each child containing those things he is allergic to, as determined by his skin tests. Small amounts of the extract are injected under the skin by a tiny needle, which hardly hurts, on a weekly basis—sometimes twice a week. Most children, after a few visits, come to the nurse's station by themselves. They hold up their arms and fearlessly receive an injection with scarcely a wince.

The child usually waits in the office for fifteen to thirty minutes after the allergy injection is given. Any reaction that may occur is noted on the child's chart. If there is no reaction, the amount of extract given the next time is increased until an adequate level for maintenance is obtained. The maintenance dosage may be given less frequently, possibly every ten days to two weeks. Some physicians give each extract separately. However, multiple injections are necessary, which is always a disadvantage in dealing with children. I prefer to combine the extracts into one solution. Recently, emulsion type treatment has been developed. With this method only one injection is necessary every few months. A number of undesirable effects, however, may occur. This method is not recommended for children unless conventional therapy has failed.

63

A mother, even if she is a nurse, should not have to assume the responsibility of giving allergy injections at home. It could be upsetting to the child and if there is a severe reaction to the shot, proper action could not be taken objectively. Besides, all emergency drugs cannot be kept at home.

Parents always ask how long the hypodesensitization shots need to be continued. This depends on the response of the individual child. Ideally, most allergists would like to see the child symptom-free for one year before stopping hypodesensitization. Please remember the allergic response is reduced by the shots—never completely cured.

A child who has had a wonderful response to hypodesensitization therapy may all of a sudden regress to his former ways. This signifies a change in the patient's allergic picture. The patient has probably acquired additional allergies which were not previously present. This usually takes a year or more. However, in the very young child it may occur within six months. The solution to this problem is to repeat the skin tests and make a new vaccine.

Breathing Exercises

The distensibility of the chest wall and rigidity of the bony rib cage may be affected in chronic respiratory disease. These are called nonpulmonary factors. Exercises are effective when the child is old enough to cooperate—at approximately six years of age. The exercises should be practiced for ten minutes three times a day and later increased to twenty minutes twice a day. How to do the exercises is described below. If in doubt, ask your physician to show you.

1. *Diaphragmatic breathing*—The child lies flat on his back with his knees flexed (bent) and one hand resting on his chest. The object of the exercise is to completely empty the lungs. The exercise begins with a short sniff through the nose, followed by a long expiration through the mouth making an "F" or "S" sound with the lips and teeth. As the child exhales slowly he gently sinks his chest as much as possible and then the upper part of his stomach. The exercise should be repeated ten or twenty times with rest as needed.

2. *Side expansion breathing*—This exercise is done with the child in a sitting position and his back against a chair. The hands

are placed with the little fingers resting on the lowest rib. The shoulders must be kept down or forward. The exercise is begun with a short sniff through the nose; breathing out is done slowly through the mouth, first sinking the chest as much as possible and then squeezing the ribs to help expel the air from the lungs. This is repeated ten to twenty times, with rest as needed.

3. *Forward bending*—The child sits with his arms relaxed at his side and breathes out slowly while dropping his head. He sinks his chest and then bends forward until his head is between his knees. The child then gradually breathes in while raising his body so that the back, shoulders, neck, and finally the head, are in the original position.

4. *Mobility exercises*—The child stands with his arms swinging loosely and rotates the trunk to each side. He also sits or stands, alternately swinging each arm above his head, and then bends down to touch the opposite leg below the knee.

5. *Elbow circling exercise*—This exercise is repeated several times between the breathing exercises. It is done in the sitting position. The fingers are placed on the shoulders maintaining the elbows parallel to the floor. The elbows are moved in circles with the movement taking place in the shoulder joints.

ASTHMATIC BRONCHITIS (ALLERGIC BRONCHITIS)

Asthmatic bronchitis is a disease condition which may be referred to by other names by your physician, depending upon the part of the country in which he was trained. If there is any doubt in your mind, ask your physician. By asthmatic bronchitis I mean there is a chest infection, namely bronchitis, with an associated wheeze. The wheezing only occurs when an infection is present in the chest. Its presence should be suspected in children with frequent colds, recurrent or protracted bronchitis, and persistent spasmodic cough. It is particularly common during the first three years of life. The wheezing, however, will stop when the infection is treated. The section headed Bronchitis should be referred to. In addition, wheezing medicine is given. The influencing factors and the recommendations for treatment discussed under Asthma and the Allergic Patient should be considered. A large number of children with asthmatic bronchitis will subsequently develop classical symptoms of asthma. Hypodesensitization, however, should prevent such an outcome in many.

ATHLETE'S FOOT

Athlete's foot is a fungus infection that occurs between the webbing of the toes. It is more apt to occur when this area is not thoroughly dried. Desenex Powder is available in the drugstore without a prescription. Apply Desenex Powder twice a day and put on a dry pair of socks. If improvement is not obvious in one week, consult your physician.

B

BED WETTING—ENURESIS

The medical term for bed wetting is enuresis. It is hard to decide on an acceptable definition. Most physicians would agree that bed wetting represents repeated involuntary urination after the age of four years. If the problem of bed wetting should persist much beyond the age of starting school, your doctor should be consulted.

Usually there has never been a long symptom-free period. In some cases bed wetting has occurred after a dry period of a year or more. A careful history is taken and a physical examination always performed.

Bed wetting that is due to some physical abnormality will occur throughout the day and not only at night. Appropriate diagnostic tests are requested when indicated. A urinalysis should always be done. The child may need an intravenous pyelogram (IVP), in which harmless dye is injected into a vein. The dye is concentrated in the kidneys and demonstrates the outline of the kidneys, ureters and bladder. The ureters are long tubes which allow the urine to flow from the kidneys to the bladder.

In some cases a cystoscopic examination may be necessary. With the cystoscope the doctor can look directly into the bladder. To do this he passes a tube through the urethra, through which humans void. This is not a painful procedure. Only a local anesthetic is needed. Such examinations will rule out specific diseases such as infections or urinary tract abnormalities. If any congenital abnormalities are found surgery may be indicated.

The commonest causes of bed wetting are tension and emotional problems. Frequently, bed wetting will occur in a child for the first time when there is a new addition to the family, or when the family moves. In these cases the cause is obviously a feeling of insecurity and the child should be reassured. Bed wetting can also be due to frightening dreams or nightmares. If there has been a great battle over bed wetting during the day, the child may comply while awake, but at night his unconscious mind may express his true feelings.

A tranquilizer is frequently helpful. However, tranquilizers are treating the symptom and not the underlying illness. If such medication is necessary, parents should examine the relationships existing in the family.

To restrict fluids prior to sleep, to wake the child up in the middle of the night, and to punish the child can only do further harm. This is also true of letting the child sleep in a wet bed because he dislikes it. Shame and guilt should not be created in any child.

Think how the child feels. He would like to comply with his parents' wishes but he has not yet developed control over his unconscious mind. Everything should be done to improve your child's self-image without bribing him.

Some children who are controlled most of the time will wet when they are extremely excited, or laugh suddenly. This is normal. Do you remember starting out for a job interview and going to the bathroom three or four times the hour before? Certainly, such a child in the school system must be allowed to go to the bathroom when necessary. If the teacher does not understand, ask your physician to call and explain the situation to her.

Some children know they need to go, but are so involved in playing that they cannot give it up, and keep stalling. If this occurs occasionally, it is normal. If it occurs regularly, parents must look at the underlying meaning, with the help of a trained professional.

Many children as they grow older will wet less frequently because the size of the bladder increases. You may help your child increase his bladder capacity. He is asked, with your help, to keep a record of the amount of urine voided, using a measuring cup. The typical child will void two to six ounces at a time. He is then asked to drink additional fluid during the day and hold his urine as long as possible. This frequently increases bladder capacity and he will typically begin voiding ten to twelve ounces at a time. If this occurs he will usually remain dry. This training process may require three to six months. Naturally, the cooperation of the child is necessary. Probanthine, a drug which helps enlarge the bladder capacity, is recommended by some physicians at the same time.

A number of electrical devices based on a conditioned reflex are on the market. They are designed to close an electrical circuit when urination starts, and then a buzzer, bell or shock wakes the patient. Most physicians do not believe these electrical devices are of value. I personally do not recommend this gimmick.

Some children are bed wetters because they sleep more soundly than others. In this case, there may be a family history of bed wetting. Sometimes this type of child will be helped by a stimulant prior to sleep. They have such an extraordinary tolerance to the stimulant that their sleep is not actually interfered with. However, if the child should begin to sleep poorly, the stimulant should be discontinued.

I have found the routine use of drugs, except for reasons stated above, to be of little value. If such drugs as Imapramine are used, the child usually reverts to bed wetting as soon as the drug is stopped.

BITES—ANIMAL (ALSO SEE CUTS)

Animal bites should be thoroughly cleaned with soap and water. I recommend Phisohex, which is available in the drugstore without a prescription. It helps prevent the growth of bacteria. If bleeding occurs, it should be allowed to continue for a short period of time as it is an excellent means of cleansing the wound. Then apply a dry sterile dressing. If the wound is large or deep, stitches may be required.

Your doctor's office should be contacted to determine if it is necessary for your physician to see the child. His nurse can tell you if a tetanus booster is necessary. The Health Department should be notified, as there is always the possibility of rabies with any animal bite. It is the responsibility of the parents to do this unless instructed otherwise. The Health Department will have a sanitation expert find the animal, and then make arrangements for quarantine. Rabies shots are not routinely recommended unless the bite is on the face or neck, where it is closer to the central nervous system, or unless the animal develops signs and symptoms of rabies. (See Rabies.)

If the bite becomes red, swollen, hot or tender, secondary infection has occurred. Consult your physician since antibiotic therapy will probably be necessary. Unfortunately, starting antibiotics immediately after the bite seems to be of little value in preventing secondary infection. Hot soaks placed over the infected area for twenty minutes four times a day are extremely valuable. (See Hot Soaks.) Infection may cause increased scar tissue and thus a poorer result.

For a better cosmetic result after the wound has completely healed, rub the scar tissue in a circular motion with lanolin for five minutes a day until it is soft, or for six months, whichever occurs first.

BITES—BLACK WIDOW SPIDER

The black widow spider is usually a docile insect and must be provoked before biting. It can be identified by an hour glass red spot on its otherwise black body. Its bite can cause abdominal pain mimicking acute appendicitis. Abdominal pain from this cause should be considered if black widow spiders are native to your area. A specific serum is available for treatment. The response is excellent.

BITES—HUMAN

The treatment of a human bite is the same as that described above under Bites—Animal, with one exception: the possibility of rabies does not exist. However, there is nothing dirtier than a human bite and secondary infection is very common.

Children before the age of two years frequently bite each other. It is meaningless; no punishment is necessary. However, after the age of two biting is not socially acceptable. If biting continues or becomes more persistent, it is a sign of an underlying psychological problem. New techniques of handling the child will have to be learned by all. Spanking the child will not prevent the problem unless excessive fear is created. If fear is instilled, poor behavior will then manifest itself in some other way.

BLISTERS

Blisters may be filled with water or blood. If they are small, they should be left alone until the fluid is naturally absorbed. A large blister may be opened by the parents. Sterilize a needle by holding it in a flame. Wash the blister and puncture it at the edge. Gently press the edge of the blister with sterile gauze to remove the fluid. If any signs of infection develop—redness, swelling, heat or tenderness—consult your physician immediately. If blisters are due to burns consult your physician right away. (See Burns.)

BOWED LEGS (ALSO SEE RICKETS)

Bowing of the lower extremities is present in almost all babies at birth. This is due to the position of the baby's legs while growing in the mother's uterus. This curving, however, is usually mild. In most cases the legs will gradually straighten out themselves, without specific correction. This generally occurs after the baby has been bearing weight (standing) for approximately six months.

In unusually severe cases of bowing, casts from below the knee for four to six weeks will straighten the legs satisfactorily. In little girls, where the cosmetic result as well as the functional may be a consideration, there is a greater indication for casts. Some physicians may honestly differ as to the necessity of casts in a particular case. This is a judgment decision. It must be remembered that in the normal development of the posture of the legs there is a turned-inward phase to the age of two years, and a bent-outward phase between two and twelve years. During adolescence there is a balancing effect with few individuals having absolutely straight legs. I would personally prefer to correct bowed legs early rather than wait too long. As the infant grows older the same treatment becomes more difficult.

BOWEL MOVEMENTS (STOOL)

A. Number Per Day.   Every baby is an individual. Some have one bowel movement a day, others one after each feeding, or even one every other day. These variations are all normal. The stool should be soft and yellow. Breast fed babies commonly have more frequent bowel movements than bottle fed babies. Their stools may have a larger water ring. If the stool turns green consult your doctor as this may be the sign of an infection in the intestinal tract. Special formulas such as Sobee cause the stools to be looser and smell differently.

B. Mucous in the Stool. Mucous in the stool may be a sign of infection in the intestinal tract. Your physician should be consulted. Sometimes mucous occurs from indigestion, or when the baby has a cold, but this judgment should not be made by the parents. Allergy is also a consideration.

C. Blood in the Stools. The commonest cause of a small amount of blood in the stool is a rectal fissure. The mucous membrane lining the intestine tears slightly, usually secondary to a hard bowel movement. This may be easily seen by examining the rectum Always consult your physician in this case. He will probably prescribe some ointment or suppositories to promote healing of the fissure. Try to keep the stool soft by having the child drink prune juice in the morning. (See D below—Constipation.) If an infant is nursing, a cracked nipple commonly causes blood in the stool. A large amount of blood in the stool may be the sign of a surgical condition of the abdomen. Consult your doctor immediately. Eating beets may cause the stool to appear red—do not confuse this with blood in the stool.

D. Constipation. One stool a day or every other day is not harmful to your baby. This does not mean he is constipated. Hard lumpy stools do not necessarily mean the baby is constipated. Only if the baby is straining and in pain while having a bowel movement is he constipated. Frequently, infants become constipated when they are changed from formula to whole milk.

If constipated, the baby should have something that will make the stools softer and looser. Prune juice that an adult may drink, mixed with an equal amount of water, is excellent. A few ounces may be given every morning at 10 a.m. Additional sugar added to the baby's water also helps. All fruits, spinach and liver help prevent constipation. Most physicians recommend these dietary measures instead of prescribing laxatives and suppositories. If drugs are used excessively the baby will become dependent upon them. He will not have a bowel movement without them. Infant size glycerine suppositories may be occasionally used. They are available in the drugstore without a prescription. Zymenol is an excellent prepara-

71

tion to prevent constipation as it is a yeast product and not habit forming. It is available in the drugstore without a prescription. The recommended dosage is one-half teaspoon at the hour of sleep for children under three; one teaspoon at the hour of sleep for children between the ages of three and six; one tablespoon at the hour of sleep for children between the ages of six and twelve. Enemas are rarely indicated and may be dangerous. Castor oil no longer has a place in the treatment of constipation. Cathartics, such as Milk of Magnesia are rarely necessary. Mineral oil should not be given to babies. If mineral oil is accidently taken or breathed into the lungs it may cause pneumonia.

Occasionally, a child may become frightened about having a bowel movement because the previous movement was hard and thus painful. Sometimes the stool may be even hard enough to cause a small tear in the mucous membrane of the anus. This is called a rectal fissure and is the commonest cause of a small amount of bright red blood in the stool. (See C—Blood in the Stool.) Parents can reassure the child that while they know it hurts, future movements will be soft because of medication and changes in the diet.

BREATH HOLDING

Babies that have temper tantrums sometimes hold their breath for such a long period of time that they turn blue. This is a frightening experience for parents. I can assure them, however, that *the child will breathe again by himself.* Let me prove it to you. Carbon dioxide, which collects in the blood stream, is the stimulus for our next breath. It is impossible for a child of any age not to respond to this stimulus. Hold your breath and note the length of time before another breath is taken. Now, breathe deeply in and out ten times and hold your breath again. In the second illustration you were able to hold your breath longer because with deep breathing you blew off more than the usual amount of carbon dioxide; thus it took a longer period of time for carbon dioxide to accumulate in your blood and stimulate your next breath. Could you voluntarily increase your best time by thirty seconds? Try it.

Do not let a baby use breath holding spells to control you. If a baby holds his breath when put to bed, do not pick him up to pacify him. Simply tuck him in, kiss him good-night and leave the room. No harm will come to him.

BREATHING—NOISY

Babies with noisy breathing should be checked by their physician. Chronic prolonged noisy breathing in the newborn is quite different from acute noisy breathing in the older child. Chronic noisy breathing in the newborn period is usually due to the cartilage in the back of the throat still being soft (laryngomalacia). It is the collapse of this cartilage as the baby breathes that causes a crowing noise medically called stridor. An infant will outgrow laryngomalacia.

Chronic noisy breathing can also be due to enlarged adenoids, and if so, tonsillectomy and adenoidectomy may be necessary. (See Adenoids. See Tonsillitis.)

Acute noisy breathing may be due to acute croup, asthma or other infections. Your physician should be consulted immediately. (See Croup. See Asthma.)

BROKEN BONES (FRACTURES)

Falls, automobile accidents and blows may break bones. Specific fractures are not discussed in this book except under the headings Collar Bone (Clavicle) and Head Injury. Out of all the falls that children have it is really amazing how seldom anything serious results. A fracture should be suspected if:

1. The child cannot move the injured part.
2. Deformity is present.
3. Pain is present when moving the injured part.
4. Lack of feeling (numbness).
5. Swelling.
6. Blueness of the skin.

A fracture itself almost never is an emergency. Call your physician and make arrangements to see him. The suspected fracture should be placed in a splint before the child is moved. A firm pillow makes an excellent support. An X ray is always taken when there has been an injury since this is the only way to rule out the presence of a fracture. Most fractures in children are reduced through manipulation, after which a cast is applied. The type of fracture determines how long a cast is necessary. Rarely is open surgery necessary. Since children have marvelous recuperative powers the results obtained are usually excellent.

BRONCHIECTASIS

Bronchiectasis means that chronic lung disease is present. There is permanent collapse of the air spaces in some areas of the lung. This may be followed by scarring of the lung tissue. The lung tissue has lost its elasticity and can no longer function normally. The first major symptom is severe bouts of coughing. Sputum may or may not be raised as children frequently swallow it. Occasionally there is spitting of blood. The child is usually underweight. A low grade fever is often present. Frequently, the sinuses become infected. As the disease progresses deformities of the chest develop and the ends of the fingers become club shaped.

Bronchiectasis may stem from untreated asthma, chronic cough or chronic bronchitis. A chest X ray demonstrates changes taking place in the lung tissue. More specific information may be obtained by installing a harmless radiopaque liquid into the bronchial tree prior to taking the X ray. Vigorous medical treatment must be employed against the underlying cause to prevent further development of chronic lung disease. The changes in the lung tissue which have already taken place are not reversible. If only one lobe of the lung is involved, surgical excision of that lobe may be indicated. Fortunately, man can live a perfectly normal life with one lung. It is important that the long-term approach be used. The child should see a physician at regular intervals so that all the advances of modern medicine can be used to help him.

BRONCHITIS

The trachea (windpipe) leads to a large main bronchus that divides into a slightly smaller right and left main bronchus, which extends to each side of the chest. An infection involving these bronchi is called bronchitis.

A. Signs and Symptoms. The major symptom is cough. It usually becomes progressively worse without treatment. The parents may be able to feel the mucous in the chest with their hands. Fever is not always present. I wish it were, as fever lets the parents know that the child is sick. It also means that one of the patient's body defense mechanisms is fighting infection. The diagnosis is established by your physician when he listens to your child's chest with his stethoscope. An X ray of the chest is usually not necessary.

B. Etiology (Cause). Bronchitis may be either a viral or bacterial infection. It frequently develops as a complication of a cold.

C. Treatment. All suspected cases of bronchitis should be seen by a physician. Specific treatment consists of antibiotic, based upon what bacteria your doctor feels is the cause of the infection. Remember, antibiotic is of no value in a viral infection. Cough syrup, antihistamines to control the mucous, fever medications, a vaporizer, restriction of milk (which produces mucous), nose drops and rest are most helpful. The suggestions made under the symptomatic treatment of the common cold should be studied in detail. Children get sick rapidly but recover quickly—often within a week's time. After a severe case of bronchitis the child may continue to cough for two or three weeks. This cough may sound particularly bad at night or in the morning, since the mucous pools in the back of the throat, when the child is lying down. As long as your physician has examined your child and knows that the chest is clear, the continued production of mucous should be of no concern to you. During this time antihistamine may be continued on a regular basis.

D. Incubation Period. The incubation period cannot be categorically stated as this depends on the specific cause of the infection.

E. Period of Communicability. The period of communicability is from the first signs and symptoms of infection until it has been eradicated. However, bronchitis is not highly communicable.

F. School Attendance. The child should stay home from school while the symptoms are acute or until school attendance has been approved of by his physician.

G. Prevention. There is no known prevention, but the common sense approach to the common cold may lower its incidence.

H. Complications.   Complications are unusual except in untreated cases where the infection may spread deeper into the chest causing pneumonia. (See Pneumonia.)

BRUISES (CONTUSIONS)

Bruises are caused by small blood vessels that break under the skin. The injury is at first red and then turns black and blue like the typical shiner involving the eye. Minor bruises need no attention. However, if the bruise is on the belly wall (abdomen) your physician should be consulted as internal bleeding is always a possibility. Children occasionally rupture their spleen located in the left upper part of their abdomen by falling over bike handles. Damage to the liver located in the right upper part of the abdomen is extremely rare. If the contusion is over a joint a fracture must be considered. This requires an X ray.

BURNS

Little responsibility for the treatment of burns should be assumed by any parent without professional advice. It is wise to consult your physician in all cases. Burns are divided into three categories.

1. *First degree burn*—the skin becomes red but there are no associated blisters.
2. *Second degree burn*—the skin becomes red and there are associated blisters.
3. *Third degree burn*—the full thickness of the skin, including the deeper blood vessels, are involved.

The severity of a burn is directly related to the degree and amount of body surface involved. Sunburn is the commonest cause of first degree burn. In toddlers it can be a serious problem, because their bodies, percentage wise, contain more water than those of adults. Second and third degree burns involving more than one arm or leg, or a more extensive body area, require immediate hospitalization. One or two hour's delay may mean the difference between life and health in such a situation. A tremendous amount of fluid is lost through the burned skin. This fluid must be replaced or shock will occur. Fluid is given directly into the patient's vein and if necessary a blood transfusion is given. Control of pain is essential. Morphine is commonly used for this purpose. The specific treatment selected for the burned site will depend upon your physician's training, the total body area involved, and the degree of burn.

Some physicians prefer to leave the burned area exposed to the air. The dead tissue is removed and antibiotic ointment is applied. Other physicians prefer to remove the dead tissue and completely bandage the burned area until a healing occurs. Skin grafts are usually required with third degree burns and scarring may be extensive. An exciting advance in the treatment of burns has recently been made with the discovery that a diluted silver nitrate solution applied to the burned area promotes healing by preventing infection. Many patients' recoveries have been made easier this way, but this technique is still too new to be dogmatic about. However, in my opinion, as more is learned about this technique it may become the treatment of choice. A tetanus booster is always given.

Infection that spreads in spite of antibiotics is the most serious threat to life in the extensively burned patient. When parents visit a burned child in the hospital, masks and gowns are worn.

A child with first degree burns should recover without too much difficulty. Second degree burns will probably provide more of a medical challenge, but the outlook is favorable. However, recovery from third degree burns involving thirty per cent or more of the body surface is guarded.

BURPING

Burping is essential for most babies to help them eliminate excessive air (gas) in their intestinal tracts. This helps prevent colic. The causes of air in the intestinal tract are:

1. Swallowed air from sucking. Prove this to yourself by sucking on your thumb. To suck your thumb it is compressed between the tongue and roof of your mouth. With each suck the mouth must be slightly opened and a certain amount of air is swallowed. Fast eaters usually swallow more air.

2. The normal digestive processes.

3. Air produced by the normal bacteria in the intestinal tract

Remember, your baby is an individual. Some babies will have to be burped every five minutes while feeding, others once in the middle and at the end of the feeding. A few babies hardly ever burp. When the baby burps a little bit of food may be spit up. Do not be alarmed by this.

C

CAT SCRATCH FEVER

Cat scratch fever is caused by the scratch of a cat. It is not unusual for your physician to diagnose one or two cases a year.

A. Signs and Symptoms. In approximately fifty per cent of the cases there is a local lesion where the scratch occurred. This local area becomes red and swollen; sometimes ulcerated and crusted. The lesion is slow to heal. Approximately one to three weeks later painful swelling of the lymph nodes (glands) near the site of the scratch occurs. These glands usaually become markedly enlarged. They are tender to touch and the overlying skin is often red. In many cases the glands will remain enlarged for weeks or months before they return to normal size.

B. Etiology (Cause). Not known.

C. Treatment. Specific treatment consists of aspiration or drainage of the markedly enlarged nodes.

D. Incubation Period. Three to fourteen days.

E. Period of Communicability. Cat scratch fever is not communicable because it is not transmitted from man to man.

F. School Attendance. Other children in the family may attend school. The affected child may return to school when he is sufficiently recovered to carry on his daily routine.

G. Prevention. Be careful when playing with cats.

H. Complications. Almost unheard of.

CELIAC DISEASE

Celiac disease is a nutritional disturbance that occurs early in life. The signs and symptoms are:

1. Frequent foul smelling stools which are bulky in nature.
2. Abdominal distention.
3. Malnutrition.
4. Retardation in growth.
5. Specific disease conditions which are due to deficiency of vitamins and minerals, such as rickets, tetany, anemia, and softening of the bones.

Celiac disease is due to an inability to absorb certain foods from the intestinal track. The diagnosis is established by the typical clinical picture and confirmatory laboratory evidence of malabsorption. The treatment consists of a special diet and supplemental vitamins and minerals. All wheat and rye is completely avoided in the diet. The patient is started on a diet tailored as much as possible to taste, but consisting only of thoroughly cooked or canned fruits, vegetables, meats, rice, eggs, and evaporated or boiled milk. If the patient does not show improvement on this diet, the milk and milk products are completely eliminated. In connection with this diet, remember that butter contains unmodified milk. The diet may be liberalized after the child is gaining weight and all the signs and symptoms of the disease have disappeared. This modified diet may have to be continued for a number of years. Your physician will be particularly cautious about the re-introduction of wheat before normal growth is complete. The only adverse side effect of eating wheat may be retardation of growth, which can only be determined by careful observation over a long period of time. I would prefer to be extremely safe and avoid wheat until growth is complete. When foods are purchased to be sure to read all the labels carefully. Avoid prepared foods and mixes if the ingredients are not clearly stated. A useful pamphlet is "Allergic Allergy Recipes" available from the American Dietetic Association, North Michigan Avenue, Chicago 11, Illinois. A recipe book is available for $1.25 (Canadian) from the Women's Auxiliary Hospital for Sick Children, Toronto, Canada. This 148 recipe collection has particular emphasis placed on food acceptability to children of all ages.

CELLULITIS AND LYMPHANGITIS

Cellulitis is a diffuse infection of the skin. It may occur around the site of a puncture wound, abscess, or boil. The skin becomes

79

red, hot, swollen, and painful. Red streaks often extend outward from the infected area. This is called lymphangitis and represents spread of the infection towards the blood stream. This is potentially serious. All cases should be seen by your physician. Antibiotic therapy will be required. Hot soaks are extremely helpful. (See Hot Soaks.)

CEREBRAL PALSY

Cerebral palsy means that there has been damage to the nervous system, with resultant involvement of the muscles. It is a broad term that covers many specific diagnoses. Cerebral palsy may be due to congenital malformations of the brain, infections of the nervous system after birth, or damage from a difficult labor and delivery. Approximately seven children out of each one hundred thousand births develop cerebral palsy. Previous masturbation, sexual experience, or death wishes do not cause any baby to be born defective. There is no relationship between something the parents did or did not do. However, there are bound to be feelings of deep guilt on the part of the parents, especially the mother. If guilt continues for more than a few months, this feeling needs to be discussed with a doctor interested in handling such feelings, a trained clinical psychologist, or a psychiatrist.

Brain damage affects the functioning of various muscles and nerves, often leading to obvious deformities. Many deformities that occur can be corrected by surgery, but the simplest treatment is prevention. Physical therapy plays a major role in the prevention of deformities. Drugs are of limited value. Most communities have cerebral palsy workshops where affected children may go for physical therapy, as well as occupational therapy. Such a workshop will probably be beneficial to the parents too. They will learn about the experiences of other parents. This helps them bring their feelings about the problem out into the open. Many children with cerebral palsy attend the public school. However, if the child is severely retarded special classes will be necessary. The most important educational aspect in dealing with the severely retarded is to teach them to dress themselves, brush their teeth, feed themselves, and in general take care of themselves. I see no reason to teach the child to count to 100 unless he will be able to reason. Some of the more

80

severely affected children should live in a special home or institution.

Since 1955 a method called patterning has been employed in the treatment of neurologically-handicapped children at the Philadelphia Institute for the achievement of human potential. This patterning is known as the Doman-Delacato System. This method has received widespread publicity and currently some ten thousand children are receiving treatment at affiliates of the Institute through out the world. Recently, ten highly esteemed medical and health organizations united to heap criticism on this practice. Many experts concluded that the usefulness of the methods had not been established and the claims were based on the tendency to ignore the natural clinical course of some children with brain injury. Analyses and criticisms of the Doman-Delacato method are certainly sufficient to make parents and physicians hesitate before allowing any youngster to undergo any treatment with these techniques. The Institute itself has withdrawn from comprehensive studies which were developed to determine more exactly the merit or lack of merit in these methods. In the face of all this the burden of proof is distinctly on those who recommend this plan.

Ways to Help Your Brain-Damaged Child at Home

This is meant to be a guide to help you as parents of a child who has been diagnosed as brain injured or brain damaged. As you well know, your child is not easy to manage and perhaps you can use some tips or some "do's" and "dont's" that will make life a little easier for both you and your child. First of all, and most important, accept and love him as much as you can. He is different from other children in many ways and because his "difference" sets him apart he needs your love and acceptance very much. Don't blame yourself or him. What has happened has happened and no one can be blamed. Feeling that it is your fault will only make it harder for everyone. The child cannot help being the way he is anymore than the blind child can help not seeing or the deaf child can help not hearing. There are reasons why the child acts as he does but we are more interested in what he does and how we can help him.

The brain damaged child must have a regular schedule. It helps him to do the same thing at the same time every day. The hardest times of the day for him are usually when he first gets up in the morning, when he goes to bed at night, and mealtimes. He should get up at the same time every morning and go to bed at the same time every night. He should eat his meals at the same time every day. If he plays outside every day he should do this at the same time. Try to stick to this as much as possible. Changes confuse him. He is much better off when he knows what to expect, and if what he expects to happen does happen. If there has to be a change tell him about it ahead of time, if you can, so that it will not be sudden and unexpected.

The child should have a room of his own, if at all possible, or at least some place especially for him where he can be alone. There are times when he needs to be away from other people so he can pull himself together and be quiet with nothing to confuse him. His room or "place" should be as simple as possible, not without color but without any fancy decorations or gadgets. Things in his room should always be in the same place so that he can easily find them. This is again a big help to him to know what to expect. The more things are the way he thinks they are going to be, the easier it is for him.

Also, he should have a fenced-in yard to play in. His judgment, as you know, is not good and he does not see things as dangerous to him. Another reason for having a fenced-in yard is to keep other children out. Too many children at one time are upsetting. He can only play happily with one or two children. More are too confusing for him and in his confusion he may hurt them without meaning to be bad or mean.

This type of child is easily upset and sometimes seems to "blow up" for no reason that you can see. If you watch him carefully you may find that everyday things that would not bother most children will set him off. It may be some little thing that his brothers or sisters do which is harmless in itself. If possible try to see that these things are not done. Another thing you might do is watch for the danger signals before he blows. This may happen when he is tired or over-excited. The thing to do at this time is to get him to a quiet place and give him a chance to calm down before he does blow. The same thing should be done after a blow up. He should be calmly removed and comforted. Fussing and scolding will do more harm than good because he really cannot keep from blowing up.

You can help your child to learn by showing him how to do

things rather than telling him. Words do not mean as much to him as actions. For example, in teaching him to put away his toys you should both show and tell him at the same time. When you do tell him to do something use simple words that he can understand and short sentences. It is not wise for parents to try to teach the older child school subjects. Unless asked to do so by his teacher it is better to let her do this sort of teaching, but you can help him to learn many things such as good habits and how to get along with other people. Here again it is better to teach him by setting examples and showing him than by telling him.

Toys for your child should be simple and as strong and unbreakable as possible. He plays better with one toy at a time but gets tired of it quickly. When you see he is getting tired of one, take it away and give him another one. Too many toys at once confuse him. You have probably noticed that he often breaks his toys. When they don't do what he expects them to do (and he does not know what to expect) he gets mad and breaks them if he can. When he does this take away the toy he is throwing around without losing your temper and keep it from him for awhile. He will learn that when he breaks a toy he will lose it and will not keep on breaking toys he likes.

Punishment and discipline of your child is quite a problem as you know. Spanking him does not work very well. It is as cruel as spanking a blind child who trips and falls because he cannot see. Perhaps the best way to punish him is to put him in his room by himself for a short time. These children need to be near the people they love and a short separation often works as punishment. This also helps to give the child a chance to collect himself and calm down. Making him sit on a chair and talking to him quietly often works. As mentioned before, taking away the toys he is trying to break and not letting him have them for awhile can also be a type of punishment. Praise him for the good things he does and never punish in a fit of temper.

If possible, mother should have a rest or relief period regularly sometime during the day when someone else can take care of the child. If she can find someone she can trust she should try to get away completely once in awhile. She will be able to take better care of the child after a break and she really needs a change like this.

Your child should see a doctor regularly and very often some of the newer drugs work very well in helping him to calm down.

In general, then, to handle your child more easily, keep his life as simple and regular as possible. Avoid excitement. (T.V. is often too exciting for your child.) Warn him in advance there are going to be changes. Don't make promises unless you know they can be kept. Try not to become angry and lose your temper and shout. The calmer you can be the better it is for both you and your child. When you become upset he becomes more upset and it is like a snowball rolling downhill. Try not to expect too much from him and don't compare him with other children of his own age. I know that it is hard to manage your child and that you have a difficult job. Also many of the things I have suggested are easier said than done, but I hope that you will try, and in trying have enough success so that you will feel it is worth it.

CHICKEN POX (VARICELLA)

I feel that most cases of chicken pox can be adequately diagnosed and treated over the telephone. It is my custom to see only those children with high fever, an enormous number of lesions, or when there are suspected complications.

A. Signs and Symptoms.   Chicken pox usually begins with a mild fever. The fever even at the height of the disease may only range from 101 to 102 degrees. Several days later clear blisters appear on a red base. This is the characteristic lesion which establishes the diagnosis. Itching is a prominent symptom. Lesions may be present for as long as three weeks. The blisters become filled with pus and then scab over. When the crusts fall off, small pock marks remain on the skin. New lesions appear while old ones are healing.

The severity of chicken pox is directly related to the number of lesions present. The more lesions, the sicker the child. Some children may only have twenty or thirty lesions; others may have hundreds. Contrary to popular belief, chicken pox is not confined to the skin. Lesions may be found in all body systems such as the liver, intestines, heart and nervous system.

B. Etiology (Cause).   A virus.

C. Treatment.   Antibiotic is of no value since this is a viral

84

infection. Rest is the treatment of choice. A dark room is not necessary. Calamine lotion (Caladryl), which is available in the drugstore without a prescription, is helpful in controlling the itching. If necessary an oral medication may be prescribed by your physician for the itching. Tempra or tylenol with aspirin are used to control the fever. (See Tempra, Tylenol, Aspirin.)

D. Incubation Period.   Fourteen to sixteen days.

E. Period of Communicability.   The child is contagious for at least six days from the earliest evidence of the disease. A healthy person can not carry chicken pox to another person. Therefore, it is alright to have friends over or use a baby sitter providing they have had chicken pox.

F. School Attendance.   The patient may return to school when the scabs have disappeared. Other children in the family may attend school, but should be observed closely by the teacher and parent. At the first sign of illness they should stay at home.

G. Prevention.   Prevention should be considered in newborn infants, in children with malignant disease and in children receiving steroids. Zoster immune globulin (ZIG) will prevent chicken pox. Do not confuse this with gamma globulin which is of no value. One attack usually confers permanent lifetime immunity, but it is possible to contact chicken pox more than once.

H. Complications.   Mild bronchitis is common; it is caused by the same virus; therefore no antibiotic is necessary. Symptomatic treatment such as cough syrup, however, is indicated. (See Bronchitis.) Antibiotic is only prescribed for secondary infection, which is not nearly as common as with measles. Secondary infection may affect the ears, throat or chest. Severe headaches and a stiff neck may indicate that the virus has invaded the nervous system, causing encephalitis. If this occurs, your physician will probably recommend a lumbar puncture so that the characteristic laboratory findings may be demonstrated in the spinal fluid. (See Spinal Tap.) Even with encephalitis hospitalization is seldom necessary. (See Encephalitis.)

CHOKING

When a child chokes on a foreign body, turn him upside down and slap him vigorously on the back. Many times the object can be removed manually from the back of the child's throat with your finger. If choking is due to a mucous plug, vigorously slapping the back helps dislodge it.

If choking continues, or the child is turning blue, take him to the nearest hospital immediately. Foreign bodies can be removed easily with the proper equipment.

Bones should be removed from all fish, fowl and meat served to young children in order to prevent choking from this cause.

CIRCUMCISION

Circumcision is the oldest and most frequently performed of all surgical procedures. Unfortunately, it has become a ritual that is sometimes performed without proper medical justification. Each baby must be evaluated as an individual patient. Circumcision is indicated when the foreskin is tight around the head of the penis. Other arguments in favor of routine circumcision include data on genital cancer, better hygiene of the penis and improved personal habits. When indicated this operation should be performed prior to discharge from the hospital nursery. No anesthesia is necessary at this time.

Circumcision is not painful. The infant's hands and feet are restrained on a little board to keep him reasonably still. The entire operation is completed in a short period of time. Afterwards, a vaseline gauze dressing is wrapped around the end of the penis, which controls the slight bleeding that occurs. This dressing falls off spontaneously when it becomes dry in twenty-four to forty-eight hours. No other immediate care of the circumcision is necessary. I want to emphasize, however, that circumcision does not mean that no further care of the head of the penis is necessary.

The mother must pull the foreskin back from the head of the penis routinely when she bathes the baby. Do not be afraid to do this. This will not hurt the baby, although it will occasionally cause harmless bleeding which needs no treatment. This prevents the skin from adhering to the head of the penis. If this should happen or if circumcision is postponed when indicated, the baby may require a general anesthetic prior to correction of the problem. This subjects the infant to an unnecessary risk.

Circumcision after one year of age may prove psychologically harmful. Young children are aware of their genitalia, and surgery on any part of the penis may be upsetting without adequate explanation, which is almost impossible at this age.

CLEFT LIP (HARE LIP) AND CLEFT PALATE

Cleft lip means that the upper border of the lip is not joined together. The defect may extend all the way to the nostril. Hare lip is another frequently used term. This defect is generally obvious to the parents the first time they see their baby and is easily diagnosed by a physician at birth. The incidence of this congenital abnormality is approximately one in one thousand births. There does seem to be a hereditary influence. If a child is born with cleft lip and there has been no family history of this condition, the chances of a subsequent child having the same congenital abnormality is one in one hundred and fifty. If there is a previous family history of cleft lip and one child is already afflicted, the chances are one in four that subsequent children will be born with a cleft lip.

When an infant is born with a congenital abnormality there is always a feeling of deep guilt on the part of the parents, and especially the mother. It should be emphasized that nothing the mother did or did not do during the pregnancy, including sexual activity, personal thoughts, or various factors related to the birth such as medication, contributed to this congenital defect. This defect is not caused by foods, medication, or dieting. If guilt continues for more than a few months, this feeling needs to be discussed with a doctor interested in handling such feelings, a trained clinical psychologist, or a psychiatrist.

Surgery is the only recognized treatment. The results are excellent. A cleft lip may be surgically repaired immediately after birth, or the operation may be postponed until the baby weighs eight to ten pounds. If surgery is postponed it is often necessary to pin the sleeves of the baby's shirt to his diaper to prevent further injury. This type of restraint may also be used when the patient is recovering from surgery.

Cleft palate is often associated with cleft lip. The incidence and factors related to cleft palate are exactly the same as those stated above for cleft lip. Cleft palate is a defect in the roof of the mouth. It must be closed to allow for the development of proper speech.

87

Surgery is usually performed at eighteen months of age. After plastic surgery has corrected the underlying congenital abnormality, speech therapy may be necessary.

Feeding a child with a cleft lip that has not been repaired, or a cleft palate, is probably the most difficult problem the parents have to face. It is advisable to feed the child in a sitting position, directing the flow of milk against the side of the mouth. The baby should be fed with a nipple if possible, since sucking will strengthen and develop the muscles needed for speech. Often a regular nipple with slightly enlarged holes will be adequate. If the baby is unable to use any type of nipple, the formula may have to be spoon fed, or a special syringe used. I believe, when a child so affected is left with a visual scar, it is a good idea to teach him to assume an aggressive role and a sense of leadership. This may be accomplished, for example, by encouraging the child to excell in a particular sport so that he will gain the respect of his playmates, regardless of his scars.

CLUB FOOT

Club foot is characterized by turning in of the entire foot. The heel is drawn up and the forefoot is deviated inwards.

Club foot must be distinguished from a positional deformity, which results from the infant's flexed position in the uterus. Positional deformities can be passively corrected and a club foot cannot be. In other words, both the physician and parents can straighten the feet temporarily by manipulation. The incidence of this congenital abnormality is approximately one in one thousand births. It is more common in males. Sometimes both feet are involved.

The exact cause is not known, although a hereditary factor has been observed in approximately five per cent of all cases. X rays of the feet are not necessary as the deformity is obvious at birth.

Treatment should be started preferably within the first week of life. Early treatment consists of applying casts repeatedly to the foot until it is straight.

Another method of treatment involves use of the Denise-Browne splint. This is a metal horizontal bar to which two foot plates are attached. The feet are then strapped to the plates which are gradually turned over a period of time to correct the deformity. However, once the deformity is corrected, the Denise-Browne splint must be used with shoes mounted on it for approximately another six months. This is hard on most infants because of the length of time required for correction of the deformity. Even though I prefer casts, the results are excellent with both methods of treatment. If treatment is persistently delayed, surgery may become necessary, without the desired functional results.

COLDS, COMMON; CORYZEA, UPPER RESPIRATORY INFECTION (URI)

The commonest cause of illness among children, as well as adults, is the common cold. Some physicians refer to the common cold as a URI (Upper Respiratory Infection) or use the medical term "coryzea." Colds occur more frequently during the first six years of life.

A. Signs and Symptoms.   Since everyone has had a cold from time to time, most symptoms can be described by adults without difficulty.

The local manifestations are sneezing, nasal discharge, and nasal obstruction. The discharge is watery at first, but becomes yellow or green in color if secondary infection occurs. The area around the nostrils often becomes red with associated crusts. Mouth breathing is common.

The generalized symptoms include restlessness, tiredness, and loss of appetite. Fever is not always present. However, fever may be slightly elevated, or may be in the 103 to 104 degree range. Vomiting and diarrhea are common. Generally speaking, the constitutional symptoms are more pronounced in the younger child— the local symptoms in the older child.

A slightly raised rash very similar to measles may be present when the cold is caused by the coxsackie virus. Lesions similar to chicken pox, except that they are much smaller in size and usually fewer in number, may be present when the cold is caused by an ECHO virus.

A doctor seeing a child with a cold may occasionally want to do confirmatory laboratory work. A blood test helps him confirm the presence of a viral infection, and helps rule out complications. A urinalysis rules out a kidney infection. If a cough is present, and

89

unusually severe or persistent, a chest X ray may also be indicated.

B. Etiology (Cause).   A cold is caused by a virus. Many types of viruses have been incriminated and more are suspected. The names of recently isolated viruses include the adenovirus, coxsackie virus and the ECHO virus (Enteric Cytopathogenic Human Orphan).

Many parents ask me "why do you get a cold?" This question has many sides. Defense mechanisims help us fight infection. Examples of universally understood defense mechanisms are an adequate blood count and a balanced diet that provides our bodies with the necessary building blocks to resist infection. Altered body functions that occur in chronic diseases such as asthma are also important. In addition, there are defense mechanisms such as our level of gamma globulin which only the physician can fully appreciate. (See Hypogammaglobulinemia.) Other body defense mechanisms exist that neither the layman nor the doctor can understand because they had not been discovered by medical science at the time this book was published. Colds occur when our body defense mechanisms have failed us. (See also Colds—Prevention.)

C. Treatment.   Most physicians believe that parents should assume the responsibility for starting the symptomatic treatment of a common cold by themselves. Exceptions, in my opinion, include a child appearing unusually sick, and with sudden onset of fever of 103 or more degrees. Of course if a child does not completely recover in two or three days, or does not show marked improvement, he should certainly be examined by his physician. It may not be late enough, however, in the course of an illness for your doctor to make a definite diagnosis. If a child is checked too early, objective findings may not be found on physical examination. However, I would prefer to be cautious, particularly in a child under one year of age, and check the same child twenty-four hours later if necessary to establish a definite diagnosis. Treatment usually results in a favorable outcome. The average duration of a cold is one to two weeks.

Below are detailed instructions. *Please read the entire plan twice before taking action:*

Give aspirin for fussiness, irritability and fever. Providing the patient is not markedly underweight, the following dosages may be safely given:

1. For an infant *less than* six months of age, give one-quarter of a baby aspirin every four to six hours.

2. Up to one year of age, give one-half a baby aspirin every four to six hours.

3. For a child one year of age or older, give one baby aspirin per year of age, *up to the age of five, every four hours.* Thereafter, one adult aspirin may be given every four hours. (See Aspirin.) Baby Bufferin in the same dosages may be substituted for aspirin.

Other medications for fussiness, irritability and fever are available, such as tempra and tylenol. I usually recommend that tempra or tylenol be given in addition to aspirin as the combination is more effective. Tempra and tylenol are not salicylates like aspirin, and therefore their mode of action is different. These drugs are available in your drugstore without a prescription.

The recommended dosage of tempra is:

AGE	DROPS	SYRUP
Under one year of age	0.6 cc	one-half teaspoon
One to three	0.6—1.2 cc	one-half to one tsp.
Three to six	1.2 cc	one teaspoon
Six to twelve	2.4 cc	two teaspoons

Tempra is administered three to four times daily, as needed. Please note the *difference* in the *dosage* between the *syrup* (elixir) and the *drops*.

The recommended dosage of tylenol is:

AGE	DROPS	SYRUP (ELIXIR)	TABLETS
Under one	0.6 cc	½ teaspoon	not indicated
One to three	0.6 cc to 1.2 cc	½ to 1 teaspoon	not indicated
Three to six	1.2 cc	one teaspoon	not indicated
Over six	use the syrup	two teaspoons	½ tablet

Tylenol is administered three to four times daily as needed. Please note the *difference* in the *dosage* between the *syrup* (elixir) and the *drops*.

If the above medications do not control the fever adequately, the child should be sponged with cold water and alcohol. A simple method of doing this is to fill the bathroom basin with cold water and add a half bottle of rubbing alcohol. Dunk a bath towel in this solution, wring it out and wrap it around your child. When the

91

towel is warm, dip it in the solution again and rewrap the child. Doing this for twenty to thirty minutes will usually lower the fever a degree or two. A rapid way of doing this in an emergency is to take a cold shower with your child. Some physicians prefer to use tepid water with or without alcohol.

For children who do not respond to the above measures, or have an extremely high temperature, a shot is available from your physician that will bring down the fever within thirty minutes. This is truly a miracle drug. However, this medication cannot be used indiscriminately.

Chills and fever occasionally occur. When the child is cold pile blankets on him and when he is hot remove them. This may become quite a nuisance, but it is something the child has no control over. I want to emphasize that the severity of a cold cannot be evaluated by the amount of fever. Many children can be seriously ill without fever. Fever is good because it lets me—and the parents —know that the baby is sick. It also means that the baby is using a natural defense mechanism to fight infection.

Use nose drops for obstruction to the nasal passages. One quarter per cent Neo-Synephrine is available in the drugstore without a prescription. The recommended dosage is:

> For children less than one year of age, one drop in each nostril three or four times a day.
> For older children, two or three drops in each nostril three or four times a day.

There are many other nose drops which are equally effective, some of which require a prescription. Each physician develops his favorite medications over a period of time. If the parents prefer to use their doctor's favorite nose drops, that is fine. I would suggest, however, that the parents keep some kind of nose drops at home in their medicine cabinet at all times.

If a child fights the administration of nose drops vigorously, and must be held down by his parents, I would not make a major issue of it.

CAUTION: Nose drops used excessively for prolonged periods cause a rebound effect. The obstruction to the nasal passages becomes worse.

92

A nasal aspirator sometimes works wonders in infants when the nose is obstructed due to mucous. This is a squeeze rubber bulb with a little glass tip in its end. The glass tip is inserted into the nose: prior to its insertion the rubber ball is squeezed. As the rubber ball expands it sucks out the mucous.

Antihistamines are extremely helpful in controlling the bothersome symptoms of mucous. There are over a hundred antihistamines on the market. Obviously, if any one of these drugs provided the complete answer, fewer would be available. An interesting fact about antihistamines is that the patient may develop a resistance to a particular antihistamine after prolonged use and still respond to another antihistamine.

For the purpose of being able to hang your hat on something, Triaminic Syrup is available over the counter—which means without a prescription. The dosage of Triaminic Syrup is as follows:

1. Under six months of age, an eighth of a teaspoon may be given *four times a day.*
2. A six month old baby may be given one-quarter of a teaspoon *four times a day.*
3. Children one to six, one-half teaspoon every four hours.
4. Children six to twelve, one teaspoon every four hours.

Triaminic concentrate is available to make administration easier for the baby, but this form of the drug requires a prescription.

Antihistamine occasionally causes excessive drowsiness. If this occurs, cut the dosage in half.

Elevating the head of an infant by placing a pillow under the mattress helps control any mucous dripping down into the back of the throat.

Eliminate or reduce the intake of milk as it encourages mucous. Use weak tea, Jell-O water, Coca Cola, or ginger ale as temporary substitutes.

For mild coughs, which are not chesty in nature, use a cough medication which is available in the drugstore without a prescription. Ask your pharmacist to recommend one to you. Be sure to ask him about the proper dosage. If the cough sounds severe, is deep or not relieved by medication, consult a physician. Stronger cough preparations are available with a prescription.

Use a vaporizer at night if the child is congested and having difficulty sleeping. It is probably not necessary during the day. Medicine added to the water in the vaporizer is of no medicinal value. It is the humidity that counts. Three types of vaporizers are on the market today: (1) A hot humidifier which is electric and produces warm humidified air, more commonly known as the old-fashioned steam or croup kettle; (2) A cold humidifier which is electric and produces cold humidified air; (3) An ultrasonic vaporizer which is definitely superior because of the fine dense mist rapidly and consistently produced that delivers more moisture to the patient's airway. However, its cost and special care rule out adaptation for regular home use at this time, but it is available in most hospitals.

Since each child is an individual, some will respond better to a cold humidifier than a hot humidifier, or vice versa, but in general I recommend a cold humidifier because additional heat is not generated.

Be careful not to place a vaporizer too close to the patient since he could accidently pull it over, injuring himself. Creating some type of tent to concentrate the vapor makes it more effective, but this is not always necessary. If you do not have a vaporizer, steam the child in the bathroom for twenty minutes four times a day by turning on all the hot water spigots. Boiling water on a hot plate is another substitute. This arrangement, however, should not be continued beyond the parents' bedtime because of a possible fire hazard.

Mouth washes for gargling are helpful if your child is old enough. My favorite preparation is S.T.37, which is available in the drugstore without a prescription. Dilute S.T.37 with an equal amount of water and gargle two to four times a day when necessary for relief of throat pain. In the younger child use Chloraseptic spray which is available in the drugstore without a prescription. Spray the back of the throat with two squirts four times a day.

A few years ago many medical educators taught that the intake of large amounts of vitamin C would prevent or cure the common cold. This theory is not believed by most physicians today.

A well advertised myth fostered by the parents' desire to do something positive concerns chest rubs. Rubbing the chest with medication is of no value. Chest rubs do not help loosen the cough or dry up the mucous. They cannot penetrate the skin. As a matter of fact, chest rubs may be irritating to certain children.

A child sick with a cold should remain indoors, unless it is extremely warm outside. Certainly they should be kept out of the wind because wind has a tendency to chill one part of the body more than another. The usual household temperature to which the child is accustomed should be maintained. Do not turn up the heat or turn off the air conditioning. When a child has a cold it is probably best to keep the window closed at night, but certainly the room can be aired out during the day.

Years ago additional bed rest provided the best treatment for the common cold. It still does, but unfortunately it is commonly forgotten today. I am often asked, "How do I keep my child in bed?" This is a difficult question, but I have a few suggestions. By rest I mean quiet. Therefore, if your child will be happy and content looking at a book, sitting on the couch or watching television, this is satisfactory. Certainly, the child who has a cold should be kept off the floor where it is liable to be drafty. It may be that the mother is going to have to pretty much entertain the child a great deal. Children's dependency needs increase during any illness.

The appetite will definitely decrease and the child has a right to be fussy and irritable in spite of treatment. Many children will not want to take solid food. Whatever they want to eat may be given. The main consideration is that children take an adequate amount of fluid, as their bodies are composed of more fluid than the bodies of adults, on a percentage basis. As stated previously, milk produces mucous and is best avoided. Coke, ginger ale, weak tea and liquid Jell-O are fine. Don't forget the use of water unless there has been vomiting. Do not force the child to drink unless he is becoming dehydrated, and if that is the case, your doctor certainly needs to be consulted. Dehydration is discussed under the heading Acidosis.

No specific antibiotic will cure a cold since it is a viral infection. Antibiotics are used to combat secondary infection caused by bacteria and sometimes in an effort to avoid complications in an allergic child, a debilitated child, or a child with congenital heart disease.

95

Many parents who follow my advice religiously and bring their children to my office when it is obvious that they need to be seen, say: "I bring my child all the time, Dr. Henderson. My neighbor down the street never seeks medical attention when her child is sick. Am I doing something wrong?" Let me reassure these parents that they are doing nothing wrong. The person who ignores medical problems will ultimately be in serious trouble. I have seen more than one child dead on arrival at the hospital emergency room because of ignorance or denial. Do not create medical emergencies requiring heroic treatment when early detection and treatment is available. Medicine is not practiced on a statistical basis. If a child becomes a statistic he may be dead.

D. Incubation. The incubation period is short, probably twelve to forty-eight hours.

E. Period of Communicability. The cold virus is commonly spread by coughing. The affected person is probably contagious for the first forty-eight hours.

F. School Attendance. Many parents send their children to school with a cold, providing there is no fever and the symptoms are mild. As a rule, most doctors would agree with this. I want to emphasize, however, that too many children go to school with fever of 101 degrees and severe symptoms. I personally know of many children who have gone to school while on antibiotic for complications of a cold. I do not feel that this is in the best interest of the child. It is not fair to the other children in the school either.

G. Prevention. There is no satisfactory prevention for the common cold. The immunity that the child develops afterwards lasts for no more than a month. Isolation of patients and quarantine of contacts are impossible. Sterilization of the air and the wearing of masks is of no value. The liberal use of common sense and understanding the following possible predisposing factors are important in avoiding some colds:

1. Individual susceptibility.
2. Teething.
3. Allergic factors such as dust inhalation.
4. Diseased tonsils and adenoids.
5. Poor nutrition.
6. Overwhelming exposure to an infecting agent

Scientific studies have demonstrated that exposure to a cold environment, despite popular belief, does not increase the susceptibility of man to infection with common cold viruses.

Many parents ask, "Should I prevent visitors with colds from coming in when there are small children in the house?" I do not think this is necessary from a practical standpoint as the small child can be kept away from visitors if the cold is really severe.

As to psychological factors affecting the common cold, they most certainly do. It has been proven that major emotional upset can lower a person's resistance.

H. Complications. Complications due to a secondary bacterial invasion are frequent. When they occur the patient usually develops additional symptoms. The fever may suddenly rise, the cough may get progressively worse, or he may complain of earache. Your child should see a physician if complications are suspected. The common complications are ear infections, swollen glands (particularly in the neck), laryngitis, bronchitis, pneumonia, and sinusitis. These illnesses are discussed under separate headings in this book. Remember that the commonest cause of vomiting is the common cold, and that children affected frequently have loose stools. IMPORTANT: There is no such animal as a chronic or constant cold—this is the sign of allergy.

COLD SORES, FEVER BLISTERS, HERPES SIMPLEX, HERPETIC STOMATITIS, TRENCH MOUTH

Cold sores are characterized by small transparent blisters on a red base, which are accompanied by itching and burning. The above names are synonymous. The blisters quickly rupture, leaving small ulcerations which become covered with greyish-white material. Occasionally bleeding occurs from these ulcerations. The lesions may be located on the side of the gums, lips, mouth, or tongue. They frequently follow a cold.

Cold sores are caused by a virus. No specific therapy is available. If the lesions are external Blistex applied four times a day may be of value. This is available in the drugstore without a prescription. Separate eating utensils are recommended. The condition will usually disappear spontaneously in eight to fourteen days. However, if the child is in pain, your physician should be consulted. A local anesthetic applied to the lesions prior to eating may help the child drink adequate amounts of fluid to prevent dehydration. If dehydration is ever suspected see your physician as soon as possible. (See Acidosis.)

COLIC

Colic has many connotations to parents and doctors. I am talking about the baby who is irritable, fussy and fretful for prolonged periods of time, long enough to upset the mother and the rest of the household. The colicky baby has symptoms suggestive of abdominal pain. He cries vigorously. His hands are frequently clenched tight. His legs may be continually drawn up on his abdomen until he suddenly stretches them out. The infant's hands and feet may be cold and moist. They may have a bluish, mottled appearance. Vomiting, burping and passing of gas are other common symptoms.

Do not confuse the colicky baby with the normal fretful periods of babies. All babies have certain periods of the day in which they are fretful. They will be sucking a great deal, screaming or drawing up their knees. This happens even when they are adequately fed, loved, and the diapers are dry. This is normal, newborn activity. It is their way of communicating and relieving tension.

Colic is a symptom. Other symptoms besides colic occur if a serious disease is present. Common causes of this symptom are: underfeeding, overfeeding, improper feeding techniques, intolerance to food—particularly orange juice—and excessive burping. Parental anxiety, insecurity and family tensions may aggravate the symptoms. Colic in most babies is a perfectly normal reaction of a well baby. Colic does not harm the baby nor interfere with normal growth and development. Interesting enough, I have rarely seen colic in Negro babies; I know it occurs, but the symptom seems to be ignored, to the benefit of all. Fortunately, many colicky babies outgrow their problem by three months of age, and those who become colicky after that time seem to be affected less.

There is no sure cure for colic. If your baby has colic you may try almost anything. A pacifier is most useful. Sometimes a hot water bottle is helpful, but be sure not to burn the baby. Paregoric works very well. In some states, a small amount may be purchased from the druggist without a prescription. *The dosage of paregoric is one-half drop per pound of baby weight four times a day.* Such small amounts are not addicting under any circumstances. Most useful remedies for colic require a prescription since they contain some type of sedation such as phenobarbital and something to relax the stomach. They are perfectly safe to use and in the dosage required not habit-forming. The only side effects may be excessive sleepiness, in which case the dosage can be slightly reduced. Ask your physician for his favorite remedy.

If a colicky baby continues to get on the parents' nerves and makes them tense, they should ask their physician to prescribe a tranquilizer for them, even though their reaction to this continued commotion is perfectly normal.

COLLAR BONE (CLAVICLE)—FRACTURED

Fracture of the clavicle (collar bone) occasionally occurs in a difficult labor and delivery. Your physician may hear it snap. Fortunately, this does not hurt the baby. The infant is usually unable to move the arm normally on the same side as the fracture. On physical examination the actual fracture may be felt, since the collar bone is not protected by muscle or fat to any degree. The diagnosis is confirmed by X ray. Treatment consists of the application of a figure-8 elastic bandage for approximately three weeks. The results are excellent. No permanent damage is to be expected.

In older children fractures of the clavicle usually result from breaking a fall with an outstretched hand. The major symptom is the inability to raise the hand above the level of the shoulder. Diagnosis and treatment is the same as outlined above. Surgery is not necessary.

CONGENITAL HEART DISEASE

Do not make an invalid of a child with congenital heart disease. Permit him, with parental guidance, to set reasonable limits on physical activity. Let the child do those things that he is capable of doing. There is no reason why such a child should be automatically prohibited from riding a bike or playing baseball. He will soon learn how to adjust to the work load that his heart can carry.

The major signs and symptoms of congenital heart disease *in infants* are:

1. Shortness of breath.
2. Difficulty with feeding.
3. Choking spells.
4. Increased heart rate.
5. Heart murmurs.
6. Blueness of skin.
7. Failure to gain weight.
8. Recurrent respiratory infections.

The major signs and symptoms of congenital heart disease *in older children* are:

1. Shortness of breath.
2. Poor physical development.
3. Recurrent infections in the lungs.
4. Heart murmurs.
5. Blueness of skin (cyanosis).
6. Squatting.
7. Elevated blood pressure.
8. Rounding of the fingers and toes (clubbing).
9. Decreased exercise tolerance.

The diagnosis of congenital heart disease is made by:

1. An adequate history and physical examination.
2. Appropriate diagnostic tests when indicated.

These diagnostic tests may include one or more of the following:

1. *X ray and fluoroscopy* which provides direct observation as to the size, position and contour of the heart.
2. *Electrocardiogram* which measures the electric potential of the heart muscle.
3. *A complete blood count.* There may be an increase in hemoglobin in an effort to carry more oxygen.
4. *Special X-ray procedures.* Angiocardiography in which a harmless dye is injected into the patient's vein and passage of the dye through the heart is recorded by means of X ray.

5. *Cardiac catheterization.* A small plastic tube is threaded through a vein directly into the heart. Samples of blood are withdrawn from the various heart chambers and the oxygen content analyzed. The pressure in the heart chambers is also recorded. The analysis of this information leads to an exact anatomical diagnosis. All other tests, except special X-ray procedures in some cases, lend only supportive evidence to your physician's judgment.

Congenital heart disease is divided into two broad classifications:

1. *Cyanotic.* There is blueness (lividness) of the skin from imperfectly oxygenated blood.
2. *Acyanotic.* There is no blueness since adequate oxygenation of the blood stream is being maintained.

Complications of Congenital Heart Disease

1. Congestive Heart Failure. If the heart is not strong enough to meet the work load placed upon it, congestive heart failure results. *The signs and symptoms of congestive heart failure are:*

1. Shortness of breath.
2. Difficulty in breathing while lying down.
3. Swelling of the feet.
4. Blueness (Cyanosis).
5. Enlargement of the liver.
6. Enlargement of the heart as demonstrated by physical examination or X ray.
7. Increased heart rate.
8. Abnormal rhythm.

Treatment includes sedation, restriction of salt intake, rest, a diuretic which helps the kidneys get rid of fluid accumulation, oxygen when necessary, and digitalis. Digitalis safely increases the efficiency of the heart muscle. The heart is a great muscle that usually responds dramatically to this wonderful drug. It may be used safely for many years.

2. Subacute Bacterial Endocarditis. This is a bacterial infection that usually starts at the site of impaired blood flow, and involves the inner muscle of the heart and/or arteries. In children this may follow the extraction of teeth, tonsillectomy, adenoidectomy, and other operative procedures. Therefore, children with congenital heart disease must receive prophylactic (preventive) penicillin therapy prior to surgery. Treatment of this rare complication consists of massive doses of antibiotic for a minimum of six weeks. The bacteria must be completely eradicated.

3. Cerebral Thrombosis.   This is an obstruction to the flow of blood in the brain. This rare complication is more apt to occur in cyanotic congenital heart disease because there is an increase in the viscosity of the blood. The outlook depends upon the area affected and the size of the thrombosis. Generally, the possibilities for survival are poor, since the underlying condition may precipitate further trouble.

Frequently asked questions:

Q. How long will my child live? What is the outlook? Will my child lead a normal useful life? Will my child have a shorter life span than normal?

A. The answer to these questions will depend upon the degree of the specific defects and their affect on the individual child. For example, if there is a hole between the chambers of the heart, how large is it? Has heart failure been present?

Q. Does a heart murmur always mean congenital heart disease is present?

A. No. Murmurs of congenital heart disease are usually present from birth. However, the normal functional or physiologic murmur is much more common. (See Heart Murmurs.)

Q. Will my child need open heart surgery?

A. As to the specific indications for surgery, each case must be individualized and correlated with the patient's clinical course. An attitude of guarded optimism should be adopted. Sudden death from congenital heart disease is rare.

Q. At what age is open heart surgery performed?

A. Open heart surgery can be done at any age, but the more the child weighs the easier the procedure becomes technically.

Q. Is added rest needed?

A. Usually not unless congestive heart failure is present.

Q. How often should my child be checked by his physician?

A. Electrocardiograms and chest X rays are repeated on a regular basis—usually every six to twelve months.

Q. Should my child be immunized?

102

A. The usual immunization program is carried out in children with congenital heart disease, except under the most unusual circumstances.

CONTACT DERMATITIS

Contact dermatitis is a skin rash caused by contact with a substance to which the patient is allergic. The major symptom is itching. The rash is red and raised. The treatment is essentially the same as that described under Eczema. The best prevention is avoiding the particular substance to which the child is allergic. Poison ivy is a well known example. (See Rashes—Poison Ivy.)

CONVULSIONS

A convulsion is a frightening experience. Try to stay calm for the childs' benefit.

When a seizure occurs, emergency measures must be administered at home while one member of the family calls the doctor. The physician will give any special instructions to the family that are indicated and make arrangements to see the child immediately.
The emergency measures are:

1. Keep the child from biting his tongue. This may be done by keeping his jaws separated with a spoon or piece of wood.
2. If fever is present, do everything possible to bring it down. Jump in a cold shower with the child and give him aspirin rectally. A five-grain aspirin suppository may be safely given to a two year old child in an emergency. If the child is one year of age, cut the suppository in half; six months of age, cut the suppository in quarters.
3. Give some type of sedation if available. If the child has had previous convulsions, the parents probably have on hand some suppositories for just this purpose.

Epilepsy is a nonspecific term that indicates disease is present in the nervous system. The term is gradually being replaced by referring to it as a convulsive disorder to avoid the unnecessary stigma attached to the disease based upon ignorance. A symptomatic convulsive disorder indicates that the exact cause of the convulsion is known. An idiopathic convulsive disorder indicates that the exact cause of the convulsion is not known. A convulsive disorder is characterized by fits of convulsions that end with loss of consciousness. The diagnosis is established by a careful history, physical examination, and laboratory studies. The following laboratory studies are generally indicated.

1. Complete blood count.
2. A blood sugar analysis.
3. Blood calcium and inorganic phosphorous analysis.
4. Urinalysis, including a test for phenylketonuria (See Phenylketonuria.)
5. Skull X rays.
6. Electroencephalogram (brain wave) (EEG). This is similar to an electrocardiogram. The electrical discharges of the brain are recorded on paper by the use of harmless electrodes. One point to remember is that anticonvulsant medication is never discontinued prior to doing an electroencephalogram or other diagnostic procedures. This test, however, has its limitations. Twenty per cent of known epileptic patients have normal electroencephalograms and twenty per cent of patients with abnormal electroencephalograms do not have a convulsive disorder.
7. Spinal (lumbar) tap. (See Spinal Tap.)
8. Special studies such as injecting air into the brain, or dye into the blood supply, and taking appropriate X rays or surgical exploration of the brain are never done unless a morbid process is suspected, such as a tumor.

The commonest causes of convulsions in the newborn are birth injury, congenital defects of the brain, and meningitis.

High fever triggering a convulsion (febrile convulsion) is the commonest cause between six months and two years of age. Between two and six years of age the cause of most convulsions is not known (idiopathic convulsive disorder.) However, febrile convulsions are not uncommon.

Grand mal seizures are the most frequent type. They are characterized by repeated shaking and rapid bending and straightening of the arms and legs, rolling of the eyes, foaming at the mouth, biting of the tongue, and loss of control of the bladder and bowels. The duration of a grand mal seizure is anywhere from a few minutes to thirty or more. The patient is drowsy for a number of hours after the seizure. A febrile convulsion is grand mal in nature.

Petite mal seizures are infrequent. They are characterized by fleeting moments of unconsciousness. An example is repeated nodding of the head. When the head nods, the patient is unconscious for a few seconds. However, he regains consciousness so rapidly that most people are not aware of the seizure activity. Petite mal convulsions are frequently discovered because the child does poorly in school and is brought to the physician for a complete evaluation.

Treatment of convulsive disorders is based upon two principles:

1. Determine the cause.
2. Remove the cause with therapy, or suppress further convulsions with proper medication.

Since febrile convulsions are usually precipitated by fever of 103 or more degrees, the best treatment is prevention. Take immediate measures to control the fever that occurs in the course of any illness. (See Aspirin, Tempra and Tylenol.) For those children who have had febrile convulsion, additional measures are necessary. The child should be examined by his physician at the first sign of illness, so that appropriate antibiotic therapy may be started, when indicated. The temperature will have to be checked more frequently in an effort to determine any sudden rise in fever which may be controlled by cold alcohol rubdowns. Sedation which quiets the nervous system so that it does not respond as easily to fever must always be on hand. Common examples are phenobarbital and chloral hydrate. Most physicians want the parents to start this type of medication when fever is present, even before they are consulted. Remember to take this medication with you on vacations, and to send it with your child when he is away from home.

Specific permanent anti-convulsant medication is usually not prescribed for febrile convulsions, unless they are unusually severe or frequent.

Parents must not become complacent about repeated febrile seizures, assuming that their child will get well by himself if his fever is controlled. A febrile convulsion may be the only sign of meningitis, which cannot be ruled out unless the doctor is consulted. I want to emphasize something that was impressed upon me during my training. Not all physicians believe this, but I feel strongly about it because of the possible consequences. *All infants who have a febrile convulsion should have a lumbar puncture (spinal tap) with each occurrence since this is the only procedure that will definitely rule out meningitis.* More than one disease may be present at a time. Remember the old saying "an ounce of prevention is worth a pound of cure." A spinal tap (lumbar puncture) is not a difficult or dangerous procedure. A needle is placed between the vertebra in the lower part of the back. Spinal fluid is withdrawn and sent to the laboratory for analysis. (See Spinal Tap.)

The drug of choice for grand mal seizures is phenobarbital. The smallest possible dose is used in the beginning. The quantity of the medication is then gradually increased until there is adequate control of the seizure activity or until minor toxic effects occur. Your physician will instruct you about these side effects. If side effects occur, the amount of medication is reduced to nontoxic levels. Then another medication is added, for example dilantin. If a particular drug is totally ineffective, one that is helpful is substituted. All patients receiving long-term medication will probably have their blood counts checked occasionally by their physician to make sure there are no adverse side effects.

The drugs of choice for petite mal seizures are zarontin and tridione. The principles of treatment are the same.

Once seizure activity is controlled, regardless of the type of convulsive disorder present, drug therapy is continued for an indefinite period of time, or at least until the patient is seizure-free for a minimum of three years. When drug therapy is finally withdrawn it is done gradually over a period of months. Rapid withdrawal of drugs may result in the return of seizure activity.

Children with a convulsive disorder can and should be allowed to lead normal productive lives. Perhaps no other disorder has such an aura of dread and mystery, and such a body of misinformation surrounding it. Most of these children can play with their friends, take part in many games and sports, and go to school. In most cases affected persons can drive an automobile; many raise children. It is time to let the non-existing ghost out of the closet. However, in some children bike riding may be more hazardous. Work out these hazards in advance and avoid as many as possible.

106

COUGH—CHRONIC

Chronic cough occurs mostly at night, or is at least worse at night. It may even be severe enough to keep the child awake. When the child lies down mucous pools in the back of the throat and then drips down. Chronic cough is non-productive in children, i.e., no sputum is brought up. The common causes are:

1. Asthma.
2. Allergies.
3. Mucovisidosis (Cystic Fibrosis).
4. Tuberculosis.
5. Chronic Bronchitis.
6. Whooping Cough.
7. Pneumonia.
8. Postnasal Drip.

An adequate workup includes a complete history, physical examination, and appropriate diagnostic tests. The treatment depends on the cause.

COUGH MEDICATION

Cough syrups help to relieve a symptom, but do not treat the underlying illness. Their main purpose is to conserve energy and allow the child to get adequate rest.

Coughing itself is a normal defense mechanism that helps raise mucous, particularly in the older child. Most physicians wish that young children could cough the mucous up instead of constantly swallowing it. Many excellent cough preparations are available in the drugstore without a prescription. Ask your pharmacist which one he recommends and the proper dosage. If the child does not respond to medication favorably within a few days he should be examined by his physician. Changing from one cough syrup to another that does not require a prescription is of limited value.

CRADLE CAP (SEBORRHEIC DERMATITIS)

Cradle cap is characterized by greasy scales on the scalp. It is frequently found over the soft spot, and in severe cases extends on to the forehead, eyebrows, and creases behind the ears and cheeks. Itching is not a symptom. The best treatment is prevention by properly scrubbing the entire scalp with soap and water. The baby's soft spot will not break under any circumstances. Use a stiff brush. A tooth brush is good for this purpose; if necessary soften the crusts with mineral oil. Fostex Cake or Cream helps eliminate cradle cap and may be obtained in the drugstore without a prescription. The directions for its use are on the package. Recurrences are frequent.

CRANIOSYNOSTOSIS

The bones which make up the skull have a small space between them called suture lines, which allows them to grow. If these suture lines close prematurely, the bony skull is unable to grow; thus, the term craniosynostosis. The growth of the brain is impeded, leading to mental retardation. This condition is curable and complications do not occur when it is diagnosed early in life. However, once mental retardation has occurred, it is not reversible. Fortunately further retardation may be prevented if the child is young enough. This is one of the many reasons why routine well-baby visits every month during the first year of life are mandatory. The diagnosis is made by your physician feeling the closed suture lines, and is confirmed by X ray. The only acceptable treatment is surgery. I marvel at the simplicity of the surgical procedure if it is done during the first months of life.

CREEPING ERUPTION (DOG AND CAT HOOK WORM) CUTANEOUS LARVA MIGRANS

Creeping eruption, known to physicians as cutaneous larva migrans, is an extremely itchy skin irritation, most commonly found on the feet, caused by the larva of the dog and cat hook worm. The hook worm enters the skin of our children who come in contact with sandy moist warm soil in the southern United States where the larva has been deposited in the feces of our dogs and cats. Fortunately, the human body will not permit this particular larva to enter into our blood stream. Therefore, it starts to tunnel under the skin, which becomes slightly raised and red. The worm continues to tunnel as much as several inches in a day, leaving behind a track.

The chief symptom is intolerable itching, which may lead to secondary infection. Treatment consists of spraying the infected area with ethyl chloride—a local anesthetic that freezes the larva. More than one treatment may be necessary. All treatments should be supervised by a physician. The treatment of creeping eruption is not an emergency and may safely wait until your doctor's office hours. Home remedies often do more harm than good and should be avoided.

Prevention consists of wearing shoes outdoors as much as possible.

School restrictions are not necessary since creeping eruption is not spread from person to person.

To eliminate the source of creeping eruption we must free our pets from worms, keep them at home, and isolate stray dogs and cats from our premises as much as possible. Droppings from dogs and cats should be removed daily. Rules for keeping dogs and cats away from beaches and public parks must be obeyed. Sand boxes should also be covered when not in use. Worm medicine may be purchased in the pet shop for your dogs and cats. Directions for its use appear on the package. Induce your neighbors to worm their pets too.

CROUP (LARYNGOTRACHEOBRONCHITIS)

The diameter of the trachea (airway) in young children may be compared to that of a lead pencil. In croup the airway becomes swollen, thus the patient has difficulty getting air into his lungs. If the swelling is marked, respiratory distress develops which is a medical emergency.

A. Signs and Symptoms.   Acute croup usually follows a cold. The onset is sudden and takes place most frequently at night. The parents may be awakened by a loud barking noise, similar to a dog barking. Do not let this frighten you as there is little correlation between the sound and the child's condition. The noise occurs because the child is forcing the same amount of air through a narrower opening. The child is having difficulty getting air in. This is not to be confused with asthma where the child has difficulty getting air out. Hoarseness is not uncommon. Frequently the patient does not have fever, but if present it usually is not more than 101 or 102 degrees.

B. Etiology (Cause).   Croup may be either a viral or bacterial infection. Some cases are allergic in origin. A foreign body in the airways can produce the same symptoms and must be considered. The history is most important.

C. Treatment.   When the onset of croup is at night parents may treat their child at home, providing respiratory distress is not present. However, their physician should be consulted the next day. If respiratory distress is present, the child's physician should be called immediately. The signs and symptoms of respiratory distress are sucking in, in the neck, between the ribs, under the rib cage and moving in and out of the nose as the child breathes. Respiratory distress makes immediate hospitalization mandatory.

The treatment of choice at home consists of a vaporizer. Either a cold air vaporizer or a steam kettle will do. Be sure not to place the vaporizer too close to the child to prevent him from pulling it over and injuring himself. Creating some type of tent to concentrate the vapor makes it more effective. Medicine added to the water used in a vaporizer is of no medicinal value. It is the humidity that counts. If you do not have a vaporizer, take the child into the bathroom and steam him by turning on all the hot water spigots. If the child's bark is not relieved somewhat within an hour, consult your physician. If there is any cough syrup available, give it to the child. Avoid milk as it causes mucous. Give clear liquids such as Coke or ginger ale. Aspirin may be given for fever. See your physician the next day even if the child seems well. Children with croup usually act well during the day but develop the bark again at night. This may go on for three or four nights. Frequently a chest X ray is recommended. Specific antibiotic is available. I personally have found cortisone to be most helpful in relieving respiratory distress by reducing the swelling in the airway.

A child hospitalized because of respiratory distress is placed in a croup tent with oxygen and humidity. His respiration and pulse are watched very carefully. If he remains hungry for air, a tracheotomy may have to be performed. This is a surgical operation in which an incision is made below the obstruction in the airway that allows for proper air exchange. Tracheotomy is a life saving procedure. If your physician contemplates this procedure, it is best done immediately without procrastination. Time is of the essence.

Young children with a tracheotomy have the habit of becoming dependent on the tracheotomy tube for sufficient air, even when they are well. It is very difficult to gradually close off this plastic tube. It is often a matter of months before the physician can wean such a child. This creates a nursing problem for the parents. However, I believe that with early treatment and diagnosis this complication can be avoided in most cases.

Croup is a very common illness, particularly in the winter. Once a child has had croup, he is more susceptible to it. Fortunately, children outgrow this problem as the diameter of their airway increases with normal growth.

Many, many cases of croup are treated adequately at home. This proves that the outlook for complete recovery is marvelous. An emphasis has been placed on the dangers of croup to avoid complications.

CRYING

Most causes of crying are temporary and not serious. Crying may be due to colic, hunger, indigestion, sickness, an open pin sticking the baby, or fatigue—which is a commonly overlooked cause. Fatigue may cause a baby to toss and turn and be restless prior to sleep. Analyze the situation to obtain a clue as to the cause of crying. What did the baby eat? Did he eat a large or small amount of food? Was he over-stimulated? Has he acted this way before? Does the crying occur every day?

Most mothers will develop the ability to distinguish between different types of cries. She will be able to tell if it is a cry of pain, hunger, or colic. This is communication on an unconscious level. Most fathers do not develop this ability. Comfort your baby when necessary, but not excessively.

How Long to Let the Baby Cry. It is impossible for a baby to hurt himself no matter how long he cries. A hernia is not caused by crying. The lungs will not rupture. Let him cry as long as he wants to, providing you know there really isn't much wrong. Once the baby is given more attention, he is encouraged to cry and act out longer the next time. The baby will win at one hour, one and one-half hours, two hours and three hours, if you allow him to. Even

111

though you are justified in feeling some irritation, try to develop a tolerance to the baby's crying.

CUTS, BLEEDING (HEMORRHAGE)—FIRST AID FOR

Minor cuts should be scrubbed with soap and water. A washcloth is fine—sterile gauze is not necessary. Phisohex liquid soap is particularly useful. Let the cut bleed a little, as this cleans the wound. Then apply an antiseptic such as merthiolate, which is available in the drugstore without a prescription. Avoid iodine since it can burn the skin. Finally, cover the wound to keep it clean. I personally use bandaids every time I can. Special types of bandages for larger wounds, such as Telfa which do not stick to the cut, are available in the drugstore. Scotch tape does not irritate the skin and makes an excellent substitute for adhesive tape. It may stick better. Even if blood shows through the bandage, do not change it as you may dislodge the clot, causing additional bleeding. Throbbing or slight pain about a cut is common. Take aspirin. Be sure to keep the wound dry while it is healing. Check on the date of the patient's last tetanus shot. If a booster has not been given within the last year get one during your physician's office hours (this is not an emergency).

If minor bleeding continues apply gentle pressure directly over the wound for approximately five minutes. This should prevent further bleeding, unless an artery or large vein is cut. When an artery is cut, the bleeding occurs in spurts with each contraction of the heart. When a vein is cut, the bleeding is continuous. When an artery or large vein is cut, apply a tourniquet to control the bleeding, while taking the patient to the doctor. A handkerchief may be knotted about a pencil. As the pencil is turned the increased pressure will prevent further blood loss. Be sure when using a tourniquet to release it every five minutes to allow blood to flow to the injured part. A tourniquet need only be released for thirty seconds at a time.

When the wrist is cut, consider the possibility of a cut tendon. Tendons allow our hands to open and close. Ask the patient to do this. Cut tendons should be surgically repaired in the operating room.

When a cut is large, gaping apart, or fat is hanging out, stitches

112

(sutures) may be required. If there is doubt in your mind as to the necessity of stitches, consult your doctor.

Sutures on the face are usually removed in five days to obtain the best cosmetic result. Sutures elsewhere are usually removed in seven days, unless the cut is deep or in an area such as the knee, where a lot of stress and strain is placed on it. Then the sutures may be left in for ten to fourteen days.

If the cut becomes red, swollen, hot or tender to touch, secondary infection has occurred. Consult your physician. Antibiotic will probably be necessary. If a cut with stitches becomes infected, some or all of them will probably have to be removed early, usually resulting in a slight excess of scar tissue. One month after complete healing has occurred, start rubbing the former wound with lanolin in a circular fashion for five minutes every day for six months. This breaks down the hard scar tissue, making it pliable, thus creating a better cosmetic result. Some individuals are prone to develop excessive scar tissue, known medically as a keloid. This is very common in the Negro race. It does not represent cancer. Even plastic surgery is not apt to produce a good looking scar under these circumstances.

CYSTIC FIBROSIS (MUCOVISCIDOSIS)

No satisfactory name describes this disease as it affects many of our body systems in varying degrees. Cystic fibrosis may mimic other diseases which affect the same body systems. Since the disease may be mild or severe, its diagnosis is difficult, except in the more typical cases. All brothers and sisters of children known to have cystic fibrosis should be tested carefully for the illness, as they may have mild manifestations.

A. Signs and Symptoms.   All of the signs and symptoms need not be present in every child.

1. Sweating which is excessive and during which a large amount of salt is lost. This may lead to heat prostration.
2. Chronic lung disease caused by abnormally thick mucous that obstructs the airways, often leading to chronic bronchitis or chronic pneumonia. These secondary infections are usually caused by the staphlococcus—a specific bacteria that is resistant to many antibiotics.

113

3. Pancreatic insufficiency, which results in chronic diarrhea with large greasy foul smelling stools.

4. Failure to gain weight.

5. Distention of the abdomen.

6. Rectal prolapse. The rectal tissue slips down out of place, and may be seen between the buttocks.

7. Intestinal obstruction in the newborn.

Different symptoms are usually characteristic of various age groups. Intestinal obstruction is common in the newborn. (See Intestinal Obstruction.) Under six months of age repeated respiratory infections, failure to gain weight and large foul smelling stools are the chief complaints. After six months of age, the celiac syndrome (See Celiac Syndrome) and repeated respiratory infections present themselves. Mild cases have now been discovered in adults who have had repeated respiratory problems. They were born with cystic fibrosis but the symptoms were so mild that it was not considered.

B. Etiology (Cause).   Cystic fibrosis is an inherited disease. It is a Mendelian recessive genetic trait. The mother and father must carry this trait in order for their children to be affected. Example: One-half of the hereditary characteristics of each child comes from the mother and one-half from the father. Draw two squares, one representing the mother, and one the father. Shade one-half of each square. Then draw the possible color combinations. One square will be completely white, another will be completely shaded and two squares will be half white and half shaded. With a Mendelian recessive genetic trait, the two shaded areas must come together to cause disease. The child represented by the colorless square would have no disease and the two children represented by the half-shaded squares would be carriers, but not affected themselves. It is estimated that one in seven hundred children born in the United States is affected to some degree or other. It is more common in the white than in the Negro race.

C. Diagnosis.   A sweat test establishes the diagnosis. The child is made to sweat profusely, usually by wrapping him in blankets. The sweat is collected on a sponge covered with plastic placed on the patient's back. Its salt content is analyzed in the laboratory. A marked increase in the salt content is indicative of

114

cystic fibrosis. There have been a number of screening tests developed to aid in case finding, but a person can still have cystic fibrosis with a negative screening test. Therefore, if the symptoms warrant testing, in my opinion the sweat test should be used. A high index of suspicion must always be maintained to make this diagnosis. *Physicians agree that all children who have repeated respiratory tract infections should have a sweat test.*

D. Treatment. The control of cystic fibrosis is a twenty-four hour a day proposition for everyone concerned. The principles of treatment are:

1. Control of the pulmonary obstruction. Many patients should sleep in mist tents, which keep the secretions loose and the airway clear. (See Colds.) Breathing exercises and postural drainage are most important (See Asthma.) Physical activity must be limited.

2. Control of the secondary pulmonary infection by the routine use of antibiotics. Carbenicillin, a new semi-synthetic form of penicillin, appears to be particularly effective.

3. Correction of the pancreatic insufficiency by adding pancreatic extracts to the diet.

4. Control of nutrition. A high protein, low fat diet with large doses of vitamins is prescribed. The intake of salt and fluid must be adequate.

Approximately twenty per cent of all children with cystic fibrosis develop allergies that require hypodesensitization injections. It is important that follow-up examinations and laboratory studies be done at regular intervals, so that the most efficient methods of treatment and management will be maintained and so that any new methods of treatment, if indicated, may be tried.

Advances in therapy have extended the life expectancy dramatically. Many individuals now reach adulthood and marry. Infertility in males, however, is a complication.

CYSTITIS AND PYELONEPHRITIS (PYELITIS)

Cystitis and pyelonephritis are acute infections of the urinary tract. The entire urinary tract may be involved to some degree. When the infection principally involves the bladder, the medical term is cystitis, and when it principally involves the kidneys, the term is pyelonephritis.

A. Signs and Symptoms. The onset of urinary tract infections may be either acute or insidious. The acute onset is more often seen in young children with few, if any, signs related to the urinary tract. The infant appears ill and the temperature fluctuates. There may be chills and even signs of a stiff neck. Convulsions occasionally occur and vomiting and diarrhea may be noted. The insidious onset is more common in older children with signs and symptoms localizing the infection in the urinary tract. There may be pain on urination, frequency of urination, urgency, abdominal cramps, and pain in the lower back over the kidneys.

B. Etiology (Cause). The colon bacillus is the organism most frequently found, but other organisms may be involved. Infections of the urinary tract are more frequent in girls than in boys because of the close relationship of the urethra through which we void, and the female vagina. Obstruction to the flow of urine due to a congenital abnormality must always be considered as a predisposing factor. Such an obstruction causes residual urine to remain in the bladder which provides an excellent culture medium for the multiplication of bacteria. A word of caution about bubble baths, detergents and perfumed soap in the child's bath: regular use of these preparations over relatively long periods of time has been reported to cause bladder irritation.

C. Diagnosis. The diagnosis is established by a routine urinalysis. A proper urine specimen for analysis and culture may be obtained by catching the urine in a clean container after voiding has begun—a mid-stream specimen. In spite of common belief, there is no need to analyze the first morning specimen.

D. Treatment. Adequate treatment of cystitis and pyelonephritis depends upon three principles. Adhering to these principles carefully will eliminate most kidney disease.

> 1. Isolation of the principal bacteria causing the infection and the selection of an appropriate antibiotic agent. The antibiotic chosen will depend upon the clinical judgment of your physician and the subsequent laboratory reports. Sulfa is frequently the drug of choice. Eradication of active infection usually requires two or three weeks of antibiotic therapy. To be certain repeated urines are examined under the microscope.

2. The detection and correction of any underlying congenital abnormalities that predispose the patient to infection. If obstruction to the urinary tract remains undiagnosed, its presence will gradually cause kidney insufficiency. Fortunately, most underlying obstructions are correctable by surgery. It is the consensus throughout the country that all male children should have a urological workup with the first urinary tract infection, and all females with the second urinary tract infection in little girls because of the unique anatomy, as discussed under etiology. Many physicians wait until the second urinary tract infection. Since the studies are not dangerous, I recommend them with the first infection in both sexes. I have found underlying obstructive disease more than once with the first urinary tract infection in girls.

An intravenous pyelogram (IVP) is performed when the acute infection has subsided. X rays are taken after a harmless radiopaque dye is injected into the blood stream, which outlines the urinary tract. If any abnormality is found, further studies such as cystoscopy or retrograde pyelography may be indicated. In cystoscopy a thin metal tube with a light at its end is passed through the urethra into the patient's bladder. The surgeon then examines the bladder wall under direct vision with the aid of reflecting lenses. After the cystoscope is in place, harmless radiopaque dye may be injected directly into the urinary tract in order to better visualize the structures. This is called a retrograde pyelogram.

3. Adequate follow-up to assure complete eradication of the infection and to prevent the development of chronic kidney disease. After the patient is apparently cured, he should have frequent urinalyses to rule out recurrence of infection. Repeated urinary tract infections, or those which become chronic, may cause damage to the kidneys, and eventually lead to kidney insufficiency. By carefully checking the urine the threat of possible damage may be avoided in most cases.

D

DIABETES

If your child has diabetes, this section should be re-read time and time again until your eyeballs ache. You, as a parent, must be able to distinguish between an overdosage of insulin and not enough insulin. This ability may save your child's life. Analyzing data from the 1964–1965 Nationwide Health Interview Sample of about 42,000 United States households, the National Center for Health Statistics estimates that as many as 4,000,000 Americans have diabetes. Fortunately, diabetes is uncommon in childhood.

A diabetic's pancreas does not produce enough insulin. Insulin is a substance formed in the pancreas, a gland near the stomach, which regulates the use of food materials, particularly sugar in the body, and the way those materials are carried in the blood. Too little insulin leads to hypergylcemia, which is an increase in the blood sugar. Sugar then escapes from the blood into the urine. Sugar in the urine is called glycosuria.

The signs and symptoms of diabetes are:

1. Loss of weight.
2. Increased thirst.
3. Increased urination.

The onset is often suddenly precipitated by infection, and the end result may be coma. The diagnosis is confirmed by blood sugar determinations. There is an increased incidence of tuberculosis in patients with diabetes.

Diabetes seems to be an inherited disease. A family history has been found in approximately forty per cent of all cases. No satisfactory test is available for identifying potential diabetics. However, if there is a family history of diabetes have your child's urine checked twice a year for sugar.

When the amount of insulin naturally formed in the body is less than is needed—as it is in childhood diabetes—the patient usually must receive additional insulin to survive. However, a few patients may be controlled by diet alone. The types of insulin available are discussed below:

1. *Regular Insulin.* This is quick acting. Its greatest effect is exerted three to six hours after injection. Almost no effect is exerted twelve hours after injection.

2. *Protomine Zinc Insulin (P.Z.I.).* The greatest effect is exerted twelve to eighteen hours after injection with a diminishing effect for about twenty-four hours.

3. *N.P.H. Insulin.* This type of insulin is prepared to be equiva-

lent approximately to a mixture of two parts regular insulin and one part protomine zinc insulin. The greatest effect is exerted at around seven to eleven hours with diminishing effects lasting twenty-four hours.

4. *Lente Insulin.* There are three types of Lente Insulin:

(a) Semilente Insulin has maximal effects six to eight hours after injection with diminished effects for fourteen to sixteen hours.

(b) Lente Insulin has an effect approximately like that of N.P.H. insulin.

(c) Ultralente Insulin has slower action with maximal effects manifested from twelve to eighteen hours after injection with diminishing effects lasting about twenty-four hours (approximately like Z.P.I.).

5. *Globulin Insulin (G.I.).* Maximal effects occur about eight hours after the injection and diminishing effects last about eighteen hours.

Insulin comes in two strengths, called U40 and U80. U80 insulin is twice the strength of U40 insulin. Insulin must be stored in a cool place and, therefore, refrigeration is necessary. Physicians will try to control a diabetic child with one injection of insulin a day. Oral medication has no place in the management of diabetes in juveniles at the present time. Diabetic children may be more difficult to control than adults because of rapid growth and development.

Diabetes is a disease about which the child must be educated. The child must be taught to give his own injections. The proper way of doing this is discussed below. Use a positive approach. Mr. Syringe is my friend. To prepare Mr. Syringe for use, wipe off the top of the insulin bottle with alcohol by using a cotton ball. Withdraw the plunger part way from the syringe so that the syringe becomes filled with air. Then insert the needle in the top of the insulin bottle and depress the plunger, thus injecting air into the bottle. This will permit the insulin to flow freely out of the bottle into Mr. Syringe. Now, withdraw the plunger on Mr. Syringe to the desired dosage. Your physician will teach you how to draw the proper dosage of insulin up into Mr. Syringe. Make sure there are no air bubbles in Mr. Syringe. Do not shake insulin, as this gives insulin bubbles. The injections may be given in four different sites on the body—the outer aspects of both thighs and the outer aspects of both arms. The site on the arm may be demonstrated by flexing the arm and seeing the bulge that occurs in your muscle. *The sites of injection must be alternated.* An injection should never be made less than one inch away from a recently injected site. Before giving yourself a shot, cleanse your skin with alcohol. Spread the skin between your thumb and forefinger to make it taut. Pretend there is an invisible bull's eye on your skin. Insert the needle at right angles. Withdraw Mr. Syringe's plunger a little to make sure no blood is obtained, and then inject the dose by pushing the plunger. If blood is obtained use another site. Withdraw Mr. Syringe and cleanse the injection site again with alcohol. Do not rub the injection site. An ideal way to get the feel of things is to practice sticking an orange with the needle and syringe.

Mr. Clock is a wonderful friend. He will tell the parents and child when it is time to eat. It is important to eat on time, even if an exciting game is going on. If the child is late for food, he may begin to have a reaction from an overdosage of insulin. *It must be emphasized to the child that when he eats less because of an infection, the insulin requirement is actually increased and not decreased,* as one might logically think.

Diet also plays an important part in the treatment of diabetes as no large amount of free sugar should be given. In some children an exact diet is necessary, calculating the amount of carbohydrates and protein required. To facilitate the use of many foods, diet exchange lists are available. Each food in any one list in the amount specified is approximately equal, in nutritional value, to any other food in that list. The parents can change or substitute one food for another, and get about the same amount of carbohydrate, protein and fat. How much of these nutritional elements and how many units from each list the child eats daily is up to his physician. He should be consulted before using diet exchange lists. Eli Lilly & Company has given such lists to your physician to give to you. Illustration 1 is a sample of a 1000 calorie diet.

The ideal weight for a diabetic is ten per cent less than normal; obesity must be avoided since it increases the demand for insulin. Moderate exercise is important.

If a child receives an overdosage of insulin, his blood sugar will drop. This may cause insulin shock. The term hypoglycemia refers to too little sugar in the blood. The earliest symptoms of insulin shock are:

1. Sweating.
2. Irritability.
3. Tingling sensations.
4. Pallor.

Memorize these symptoms. If insulin shock is allowed to progress without treatment, coma and convulsions occur. Treatment in the early stages consists of giving the patient sugar orally, such as found in Coca Cola or similar drink or orange juice. Your physician may give a small injection of adrenalin as an emergency measure to raise the patient's blood sugar. If the patient is unconscious, a sugar solution is given directly into his veins.

If a child does not receive enough insulin causing the blood sugar to remain high for a few days, diabetic acidosis and coma may result. The term "hyperglycemia" refers to too much sugar in the blood. A person in this condition should be hospitalized. Diabetic acidosis usually comes on over a period of days and is accompanied by increasingly large amounts of sugar and acetone in the urine. The treatment consists of immediate and relatively large doses of insulin given directly into the patient's veins and into the muscle. Repeated doses of insulin are given at frequent intervals until the blood sugar returns to normal. The patient's fluid balance must be carefully regulated. Fluids are usually injected directly into the veins, along with adequate doses of potassium. Your physician will also wash out the patient's stomach to prevent vomiting. If there is a precipitating infection, it is vigorously treated with antibiotics. The outlook for recovery from diabetic acidosis and coma is good, but it is a pediatric emergency.

If your child has diabetes, the above complications must be discussed thoroughly with your physician. The parents and child must learn how to distinguish between them and to give emergency treatment. I sincerely believe that these complications can be avoided if the parents will commit to memory the early signs and symptoms of insulin shock and diabetic acidosis, and take appropriate action when indicated.

121

General Rules

Measuring Food

Food should be measured. You will need a standard 8-ounce measuring cup and a measuring teaspoon and tablespoon. All measurements are level. Most foods are measured after cooking.

Food Preparation

Meats should be baked, boiled, or broiled. Do not fry foods unless fat allowed in meal is used.

Vegetables may be prepared with the family meals, but your portion should be removed before extra fat or flour is added.

Special Foods

It is not necessary to buy special foods. Select your diet from the same foods purchased for the rest of the family—milk, vegetables, bread, meats, fats, and fruit (fresh, dried, or canned without sugar). "Special dietetic foods" should be thoroughly investigated and usually must be figured in the diet.

Foods to Avoid

Sugar	Pie
Candy	Cake
Honey	Cookies
Jam	Pastries
Jelly	Condensed Milk
Marmalade	Soft Drinks
Syrups	Candy-Coated Gum

Fried, scalloped, or creamed foods
Beer, wine, or other alcoholic beverages

Eat only those foods which are on diet list.

Eat only the amounts of foods on diet.

Do not skip meals.

Do not eat between meals.

The use of the exchange list is based upon the recommendation of the American Diabetes Association and The American Dietetic Association in co-operation with the Diabetes Branch of the U.S. Public Health Service, Department of Health, Education, and Welfare.

Liquid Diets

(May be used to replace any one of the meals)

Full Liquid

Eggnog { milk.......1/2 cup........120 Gm.
         { egg........1............ 50 Gm.
Orange juice.........3/4 cup.......150 Gm.
Milk.................3/4 cup.......180 Gm.

Clear Liquid

Clear bouillon........1 cup
Orange juice.........1 cup.........200 Gm.
Gelatin dessert.......1/2 cup.......100 Gm.

Bedtime Feeding

(Only when directed by physician)
1/2 milk exchange
  (1/2 cup milk)   } will add approximately
1/2 bread exchange   } 120 calories to daily diet
  (2 crackers)

Lilly

Eli Lilly and Company

Indianapolis, Indiana 46206

PJ-0955-AMD   PRINTED IN U.S.A.   700809-46740   MARCH, 1967

Daily Menu Guide

These sample menus show some of the ways that the exchange lists may be used to add variety to your meals. **Use the exchange lists on the back of this sheet to plan different menus.**

BREAKFAST

1 fruit exchange (List 3)
1 bread exchange (List 4)
2 meat exchanges (List 5)
1/2 milk exchange (List 7)
Coffee or tea (any amount)

BREAKFAST

Orange juice..........................1/2 cup
Toast...................................1 slice
Eggs....................................2
Milk, whole...........................1/2 cup

LUNCH

2 meat exchanges (List 5)
1 bread exchange (List 4)
Vegetable(s) as desired (List 1)
1 fruit exchange (List 3)
1/2 milk (skimmed) exchange (List 7)
1 fat exchange (List 6)
Coffee or tea (any amount)

LUNCH

Meat....................................2 slices
                        (3″ x 2″ x 1/8″ ea.)
Broccoli...............................as desired
Lettuce and tomato salad...........as desired
Bread..................................1 slice
Butter.................................1 tsp.
Pineapple.............................1/2 cup
Milk, skimmed........................1/2 cup

DINNER

2 meat exchanges (List 5)
1 bread exchange (List 4)
Vegetable(s) as desired (List 1)
1 vegetable exchange (List 2)
1 fruit exchange (List 3)
1 fat exchange (List 6)
Coffee or tea (any amount)

DINNER

Tomato juice..........................3 oz.
Chicken................................2 slices
                        (3″ x 2″ x 1/8″ ea.)
Noodles................................1/2 cup
Asparagus..............................as desired
Peas...................................1/2 cup
Butter.................................1 tsp.
Banana.................................1/2 small

123

Daily menu guide

The foods allowed in your diet should be selected from the seven exchange lists on this page. Menus should be planned on the basis of the menu guide given below. Foods in the same list are interchangeable, because, in the quantities specified, they provide approximately the same amounts of carbohydrate, protein, and fat. For example, when your menu calls for one bread exchange, any item in List 4 may be used in the amount stated. If two bread exchanges are allowed, double the specified amount or use a single exchange of *two* foods in List 4. Sample menus on the reverse side of this sheet illustrate correct use of the exchange lists.

BREAKFAST

1 fruit exchange (List 3)
1 bread exchange (List 4)
2 meat exchanges (List 5)
1/2 milk exchange (List 7)
Coffee or tea (any amount)

LUNCH

2 meat exchanges (List 5)
1 bread exchange (List 4)
Vegetable(s) as desired (List 1)
1 fruit exchange (List 3)
1/2 milk (skimmed) exchange (List 7)
1 fat exchange (List 6)
Coffee or tea (any amount)

DINNER

2 meat exchanges (List 5)
1 bread exchange (List 4)
Vegetable(s) as desired (List 1)
1 vegetable exchange (List 2)
1 fruit exchange (List 3)
1 fat exchange (List 6)
Coffee or tea (any amount)

List 1 allowed as desired

(need not be measured)

Seasonings: Cinnamon, celery salt, garlic, garlic salt, lemon, mustard, mint, nutmeg, parsley, pepper, saccharin and other sugarless sweeteners, spices, vanilla, and vinegar.

Other Foods: Coffee or tea (without sugar or cream), fat-free broth, bouillon, unflavored gelatin, rennet tablets, sour or dill pickles, cranberries (without sugar), rhubarb (without sugar).

Vegetables: Group A—insignificant carbohydrate or calories. You may eat as much as desired of raw vegetable. If cooked vegetable is eaten, limit amount to 1 cup.

Asparagus	Lettuce
Broccoli	Mushrooms
Brussels sprouts	Okra
Cabbage	Peppers, green
Cauliflower	or red
Celery	Radishes
Chicory	Sauerkraut
Cucumbers	String beans
Eggplant	Summer squash
Escarole	Tomatoes
Greens: beet, chard, collard, dandelion, kale, mustard, spinach, turnip	Watercress

List 2 vegetable exchanges

Each portion supplies approximately 7 Gm. of carbohydrate and 2 Gm. of protein, or 36 calories.

Vegetables: Group B—One serving equals 1/2 cup, or 100 Gm.

Beets	Pumpkin
Carrots	Rutabagas
Onions	Squash, winter
Peas, green	Turnips

List 3 fruit exchanges
(fresh, dried, or canned without sugar)
Each portion supplies approximately 10 Gm. of carbohydrate, or 40 calories.

	household measurement	weight of portion
Apple	1 small (2" diam.)	80 Gm.
Applesauce	1/2 cup	100 Gm.
Apricots, fresh	2 med.	100 Gm.
Apricots, dried	4 halves	20 Gm.
Banana	1/2 small	50 Gm.
Berries	1 cup	150 Gm.
Blueberries	2/3 cup	100 Gm.
Cantaloupe	1/4 (6" diam.)	200 Gm.
Cherries	10 large	75 Gm.
Dates	2	15 Gm.
Figs, fresh	2 large	50 Gm.
Figs, dried	1 small	15 Gm.
Grapefruit	1/2 small	125 Gm.
Grapefruit juice	1/2 cup	100 Gm.
Grapes	12	75 Gm.
Grape juice	1/4 cup	60 Gm.
Honeydew melon	1/8 (7")	150 Gm.
Mango	1/2 small	70 Gm.
Orange	1 small	100 Gm.
Orange juice	1/2 cup	100 Gm.
Papaya	1/3 med.	100 Gm.
Peach	1 med.	100 Gm.
Pear	1 small	100 Gm.
Pineapple	1/2 cup	80 Gm.
Pineapple juice	1/3 cup	80 Gm.
Plums	2 med.	100 Gm.
Prunes, dried	2	25 Gm.
Raisins	2 tbsp.	15 Gm.
Tangerine	1 large	100 Gm.
Watermelon	1 cup	175 Gm.

List 4 bread exchanges
Each portion supplies approximately 15 Gm. of carbohydrate and 2 Gm. of protein, or 68 calories.

	household measurement	weight of portion
Bread	1 slice	25 Gm.
Biscuit, roll	1 (2" diam.)	35 Gm.
Muffin	1 (2" diam.)	35 Gm.
Cornbread	1 1/2" cube	35 Gm.
Flour	2 1/2 tbsp.	20 Gm.
Cereal, cooked	1/2 cup	100 Gm.
Cereal, dry (flakes or puffed)	3/4 cup	20 Gm.
Rice or grits, cooked	1/2 cup	100 Gm.
Spaghetti, noodles, etc.	1/2 cup	100 Gm.
Crackers, graham	2	20 Gm.
Crackers, oyster	20 (1/2 cup)	20 Gm.
Crackers, saltine	5	20 Gm.
Crackers, soda	3	20 Gm.
Crackers, round	6-8	20 Gm.
Vegetables		
Beans (Lima, navy, etc.), dry, cooked	1/2 cup	90 Gm.
Peas (split peas, etc.), dry, cooked	1/2 cup	90 Gm.
Baked beans, no pork	1/4 cup	50 Gm.
Corn	1/3 cup	80 Gm.
Parsnips	2/3 cup	125 Gm.
Potato, white, baked or boiled	1 (2" diam.)	100 Gm.
Potatoes, white, mashed	1/2 cup	100 Gm.
Potatoes, sweet, or yams	1/4 cup	50 Gm.
Sponge cake, plain	1 1/2" cube	25 Gm.
Ice cream (Omit 2 fat exchanges)	1/2 cup	70 Gm.

List 5 meat exchanges
Each portion supplies approximately 7 Gm. of protein and 5 Gm. of fat, or 73 calories. (30 Gm. equal 1 oz.)

	household measurement	weight of portion
Meat and poultry (beef, lamb, pork, liver, chicken, etc.) (med. fat)	1 slice (3" x 2" x 1/8")	30 Gm.
Cold cuts	1 slice (4 1/2" sq., 1/8" thick)	45 Gm.
Frankfurter	1 (8-9 per lb.)	50 Gm.
Codfish, mackerel, etc.	1 slice (2" x 2" x 1")	30 Gm.
Salmon, tuna, crab	1/4 cup	30 Gm.
Oysters, shrimp, clams	5 small	45 Gm.
Sardines	3 med.	30 Gm.
Cheese, cheddar, American	1 slice (3 1/2" x 1 1/2" x 1/4")	30 Gm.
Cheese, cottage	1/4 cup	45 Gm.
Egg	1	50 Gm.
Peanut butter	2 tbsp.	30 Gm.

Limit peanut butter to one exchange per day unless allowance is made for carbohydrate in the diet plan.

List 6 fat exchanges
Each portion supplies approximately 5 Gm. of fat, or 45 calories.

	household measurement	weight of portion
Butter or margarine	1 tsp.	5 Gm.
Bacon, crisp	1 slice	10 Gm.
Cream, light	2 tbsp.	30 Gm.
Cream, heavy	1 tbsp.	15 Gm.
Cream cheese	1 tbsp.	15 Gm.
French dressing	1 tbsp.	15 Gm.
Mayonnaise	1 tsp.	5 Gm.
Oil or cooking fat	1 tsp.	5 Gm.
Nuts	6 small	10 Gm.
Olives	5 small	50 Gm.
Avocado	1/8 (4" diam.)	25 Gm.

List 7 milk exchanges
Each portion supplies approximately 12 Gm. of carbohydrate, 8 Gm. of protein, and 10 Gm. of fat, or 170 calories.

	household measurement	weight of portion
Milk, whole	1 cup	240 Gm.
Milk, evaporated	1/2 cup	120 Gm.
*Milk, powdered	1/4 cup	35 Gm.
*Buttermilk	1 cup	240 Gm.

*Add 2 fat exchanges if milk is fat-free.

Once the diabetic has been adequately regulated by his physician, he, with the help of his parents, can learn how to increase or decrease in very small amounts the amount of insulin he receives, based upon a simple laboratory test determining how much sugar is present in his urine. Paper strips are available that test for sugar in the urine, and are sold as Tes-Tape and Clinistic. These paper strips need only be dipped in the urine. The color is then compared to a color chart to determine the approximate amount of sugar present. The tests are recorded as negative or "0" when no sugar is found, and positive "+" when sugar is found. Plus signs "+, ++, +++,++++" are used to indicate roughly the amount of sugar in the urine. A moderate amount of sugar (+, ++) in the urine does not of itself appear to be harmful; however, large amounts (+++, ++++) are. *The amount of sugar in the urine should be checked at least four times a day.*

Acetone in the urine must be tested for once a day. Acetone accumulates in the urine when there is an insufficient supply of insulin. Acetone in the urine may be tested for in the home by use of the Denco Acetone Powder or Ace Test Tablets. The test for acetone is likely to be positive where there is fever, vomiting, diarrhea, headache, sudden loss of weight, excessive urination during the day or night, and when the urine tests are persistently +++ or ++++ for sugar.

Any time the acetone test is positive, and increasing amounts of sugar appear in the urine, an extra dose of regular insulin should be taken promptly.

Foot care is extremely important, as diabetes is especially liable to cause circulatory disorders and infections as the child grows older. Always keep the feet clean, warm and dry. Socks should be changed daily. Avoid sunburn, iodine, heating pads, or cutting your own corns. Do not walk barefooted or take other risks which might possibly cause skin injury. Avoid tight shoes and cut your toenails straight across. Examine your feet daily and report any change to your physician.

The best rule for all diabetics to follow is "be prepared." Always try to anticipate trouble. A diabetic should wear a medallion at all times indicating that he is a diabetic. Charms are available for bracelets or key cases. A card should be carried in the wallet that identifies the child. The card should state: "I am a diabetic, please place some sugar or candy in my mouth and call my doctor, or hospital emergency room, if I am found unconscious." In adults the card would also say "I am not intoxicated." The child should keep his phone number, and the doctor's phone number, with him at all times. Teachers should be informed in school, and some special friends with whom the child plays. The special friends should be instructed to call the child's mother or doctor if their playmate feels funny.

Since diabetes is a disease for which there is no cure, but for which there is adequate control, it is important to see that the proper psychological adjustment is made. It may be necessary for the child and parents to discuss their feelings with a physician who is interested in this particular aspect of the disease, a clinical psychologist or psychiatrist.

When diabetes is well-controlled, the child can expect to live a reasonably long, full and happy life. When the child neglects to take proper care of himself he increases the chances of short- and long-term complications that can affect his vision, circulatory system, kidneys, nervous system, and resistance to infection, in years ahead. Doctors have now been encouraged by progress being made in transplants of the pancreas in adults. Faithfully following every detail of the physician's suggested daily schedule, and thus achieving good control, can make a big difference in the diabetic's day to day health, the way he feels, the leading of a normal life in every other way, and possibly the avoidance of long-term complications in later years. The child should see a physician at regular intervals so that all the advances of modern medicine can be brought to bear against this illness.

DIAPER RASH

I have never seen a baby that did not eventually develop diaper rash. Many times babies will be discharged from the hospital nursery with it. This does not mean that the nursery personnel has been negligent, but only that extra attention is needed because of the baby's sensitive skin. Diaper rash can occur in a matter of hours, no matter how frequently the baby's diapers are changed.

Diaper rash is caused by the normal bacteria on the infant's skin reacting with the urine on a wet diaper. This reaction produces

127

ammonia which irritates the skin. There is more irritation when air cannot get to the baby's bottom. Therefore, do not put rubber or plastic pants on the baby when he has diaper rash. In warm climates it is impossible to use rubber or plastic pants on a routine basis, without causing recurrent diaper rash. Inadequately washed diapers are no longer a problem with modern washing machines and diaper service. However, it is sometimes helpful to rinse the diapers in your washing machine with a product such as Diaperene Rinse granules. The directions for its use are on the package.

Some type of protective ointment should be used routinely with each diaper change. My favorite ointments are Desitin and Diaprene, which are available in the drugstore without a prescription. I like Desitin because it sticks to the skin. Corn starch, vaseline and Mennen's Baby Magic may also be used. I recently counted eighty-six different preparations manufactured for this purpose. The product that works well one week may not work the following week. The ointment that works on your neighbor's baby may not work on your baby. Often the products used must be constantly changed from week to week. In severe cases where the skin is bleeding, consult your physician so that he may prescribe some type of cortisone ointment, which promotes rapid healing. Leaving the diaper completely off the baby is also advantageous.

Amurex and Pedameth are drugs available by prescription that prevent the production of ammonia, thus helping to clear and prevent further diaper rash. The contents of one capsule is added to the entire formula supply for the day, preferably while it is still warm. It may also be given in fruit juice or water. These drugs are not harmful and may be used indefinitely.

Occasionally secondary infection occurs. Small white heads similar to pimples will be seen. Consult your physician. These little pockets of pus could provide a focus from which infection could spread to the rest of the body. In the warmer climates, fungus is often a secondary invader into the diaper area. When this happens the edges of the rash look like fine areas of peeled skin. Your physician will have to treat this since it is difficult to eliminate.

With diaper rash, sores occasionally occur at the end of the penis. Treatment is aimed at the cure and prevention of diaper rash. However, an antibiotic ointment may be applied to the sores three of four times a day. Many topical antibiotic ointments are available in the drugstore without a prescription. Ask your pharmacist to recommend one.

The results with most treatments for diaper rash are satisfactory, but prevention through constant attention is necessary. Just when the parents think they have the problem licked, it will occur again. Do not become discouraged. Keep working on the problem.

DIARRHEA—INFECTIOUS

Diarrhea is characterized by an increase in the number of stools. The signs and symptoms are:

1. A change in the consistency of the stools, to contain more water.
2. A color change, sometimes to green.
3. A foul smell.
4. Blood or pus in the stool.
5. Fever.
6. Associated vomiting.

Not all of these signs and symptoms are present in every case.

Infectious diarrhea may be either viral or bacterial in origin. There is no scientific evidence to prove that diarrhea occurs from a change in water or brand of milk. Stool cultures are indicated in some cases in an effort to isolate the offending organism.

The principles of treatment are: (1) rest the gastrointestinal tract; (2) maintain adequate hydration.

In mild cases of diarrhea—that is without a marked color change, explosive stools, fever, vomiting, blood or pus in the stools— kaopectate and paregoric, either separately or together, may be safely given by the parents without consulting their physician. Kaopectate may be purchased in the drugstore without a prescription. The precautions stated on the bottle by the manufacturer indicate that kaopectate should not be used for infants or children under three years of age, unless directed by a physician. The manufacturer must put such a statement on the label to avoid its indiscriminate use. The manufacturer is trying to make sure that all babies who need to be seen by a physician will be. Kaopectate is not harmful in any dosage. *The dose of kaopectate I recommend is:*

129

(a) One month—two teaspoons every four hours or after each bowel movement.

(b) Six months to three years—one tablespoon every four hours or after each bowel movement.

(c) Three to six years—one to two tablespoons every four hours, or after each bowel movement.

(d) Six to twelve years—two to four tablespoons every four hours or after each bowel movement.

(e) Thirteen years and older—four tablespoons every four hours or after each bowel movement.

Paregoric is available in some states without a prescription. Ask your druggist. *The dose of paregoric is one-half drop per pound of body weight four times a day.* Such small amounts are not addicting under any circumstances.

Diet restrictions are most important. If the baby is nursing and taking solids, let him continue to nurse, but eliminate the solids. If the infant is on formula, change to one-half strength boiled skimmed milk. Purchase skim milk, dilute it with an equal amount of water and boil it for twenty minutes. When the milk is cool it is ready for use. Half strength instant non-fat dry milk is equivalent to the fresh product. Skimmed milk is used because it contains less fat. If your baby is on a special formula such as Prosobee, make it half strength by diluting one can of Prosobee liquid with two cans of water.

Children six months of age or older should have their *stomachs rested for at least four hours* no matter how hungry they are, before any nourishment is allowed. Then offer small frequent sips of flat Coke or ginger ale. Avoid water as children have a notorious tendency to vomit it. Once these clear liquids have been kept down for six to eight hours, switch to one-half strength boiled skim milk. As improvement is shown in the stools increase the diet to full strength skim milk and gradually add solids, such as cereal, Jell-O and soup. Fruit is the last food to add to the diet as it has a normal tendency to cause loose stools. The principle of small frequent feedings prevents dehydration in most cases and gives the gastrointestinal tract adequate time to heal itself. Any weight loss will be rapidly regained when the child is well.

If the baby does not respond to the above treatment within

twenty-four to forty-eight hours your physician should be consulted.

Your physician should be consulted in more involved cases of diarrhea before starting treatment. Involved cases include those in which there are explosive stools, blood or pus in the stools, in which vomiting occurs more than once or twice, or in which fever is greater than 102 degrees. Various types of injectable medication and suppositories are available to stop the vomiting when indicated. The stomach should then be rested for four hours before starting the previously described diet restrictions. Antibiotics are used when indicated to eradicate the offending bacteria in the intestinal tract.

If the diarrhea or vomiting persists hospitalization may be indicated to maintain proper hydration. A child's body is composed of more water, percentage wise, than an adult's. Therefore, the child will normally require more fluid, in addition to the fluid that must be replaced because of the diarrhea and vomiting. (Dehydration is discussed under the heading Acidosis.)

Hospitalization is infrequent in proportion to the number of cases of this very common illness. Even when dehydration has occurred the response is excellent to fluids injected directly into the veins. But remember the old saying that an "ounce of prevention is worth a pound of cure." Take appropriate measures early in the course of diarrhea and prevent complications.

DIPHTHERIA

Diphtheria is a very rare disease today because of nearly universal immunization against it. Passive immunity (antibodies received from the mother's blood) provide protection for the first three months of life, and partial protection until six months of age. However, there is a slight possibility that a child may not respond successfully to routine immunization. The diagnosis, therefore, must always be considered.

A. Signs and Symptoms. White or gray patches appear on the back of the throat and tonsils. The throat is sore and fever is present. Occasionally, diphtheria may begin in the larynx causing a croupy cough, hoarseness, and difficulty in breathing.

B. Etiology (Cause). A specific bacteria.

C. Treatment.

1. All cases should be hospitalized. Diphtheria is a serious illness.

2. Specific antitoxin is given after a sensitivity test is performed.

3. Large doses of antibiotic are administered. Penicillin is widely used.

4. In laryngeal diphtheria a croup tent is used and if necessary a tracheotomy is performed to by-pass the obstruction in the airway. (See Croup.)

D. Incubation.   Two to seven days.

E. Period of Communicability.   Varies between two and four weeks, or until negative nose and throat cultures are obtained.

F. School Attendance.   The patient must remain out of school until two negative nose and throat cultures are obtained, at least twenty-four hours apart. Other children in the patient's family should not attend school until examined by their physician. School-room contacts should be observed carefully for seven days.

G. Prevention.   (See Immunization.)

H. Complications.   They are rare but serious. The heart muscle may become involved between the fifth and twelfth day as demonstrated by changes in the electrocardiogram. Nephritis may also occur. Nerve involvement may cause paralysis of the back of the throat, deviation of the eye, dilation of the pupil, or drooping of the eyelid. Fortunately, nerve paralysis is usually temporary.

DYSLEXIA

Dyslexia is a term that is being widely misused at this time. In general usage it means the inability to read. To correct the difficulty it is essential to pinpoint the cause of the child's inability to read. Dyslexia may be divided into two types: primary and secondary. In primary dyslexia there are problems in auditory discrimination where the child cannot make the connection between sight and sound. It cannot be detected with certainty in pre-school children. It is compatible with normal intelligence. Perceptual, neurologic and psychiatric examinations are all within normal limits. The primary form can only be suspected when reading achievement falls behind chronological IQ.

Secondary dyslexia results from minimal brain damage and retardation. It is associated with environmental deprivation and emotional disturbances. The diagnosis of the secondary form requires testing of visual precepts, intelligence, and language facility, together with examination of sight and hearing.

Dyslexia is not as prevalent as most people think. There are many children diagnosed as dyslexic who are not real dyslexia problems. True, these children do not seem to be able to learn to read, but the cause may be due to many other factors. There can be a general over-all lack of intelligence, there may be visual difficulties with problems not so much in visual acuity, as in focussing or convergence. There may be a lag in maturation or development. All children are not ready to read at the age of six.

If you or your child's teacher are concerned because he is not learning to read it would be wise to have a psychological evaluation to try to determine the causes of this problem. Since reading is so important in our present culture, it is advisable to do this as soon as you discover he is having difficulty, preferably in the first grade.

E

EAR INFECTIONS—OTITIS MEDIA, EXTERNAL OTITIS, SWIMMER'S EAR

A. Otitis Media.   Otitis media refers to an infection in the middle ear. The infection is behind the ear drum. Otitis media is extremely common. The peak incidence appears to be between one and two years of age. After age six there is a steady decline in its incidence.

The signs and symptoms vary from a severe cold present for a few days to high fever or no fever, vomiting, sore throat, earache and pulling on the ear. Contrary to what would be expected, ear pain is frequently not present. Occasionally the chief complaint is impairment of hearing.

Otitis media is bacterial in origin. The infection is seen when your physician examines the ear drum with his otoscope. This piece of equipment resembles a flashlight with a magnifying lens.

Otitis media frequently occurs as a complication of the common cold. The reason for this is anatomical. The eustachian tube connects the back of the nose and throat with the middle ear. In young children it is short, narrow and straight, and thus is easily filled with mucous. When this happens the normal organisms that live in the back of your nose and throat, which do not ordinarily cause infection, migrate via the plugged eustachian tube to the middle ear, causing an infection. As the child grows the eustachian tube becomes longer, wider and twisted, and the incidence of otitis media decreases.

Children with recurrent ear infections must have a careful evaluation of the nose, throat and sinuses. In children under three years of age the adenoids sometimes need to be removed to relieve obstruction to the eustachian tube. In older children, it may also be necessary to remove diseased tonsils. In addition, control must be established over any existing sinus infection.

When a child has six or more attacks of otitis media a year, allergy is the underlying culprit. Anatomically the mucous membrane lining the nose is the same as that lining the eustachian tube. Thus, the eustachian tube is full of mucous almost every time the nose is full of mucous due to allergy.

Scientific studies indicating the incidence of ear infections, after the tonsils and adenoids have been removed, after the ears have been drained, after antibiotic therapy, after nose drops and after antihistamines, prove that all of these treatments are of little value when the basic cause is allergy. However, skin testing and hypodesensitization therapy decreases the incidence by almost 80 per cent. (See Asthma and the Allergic Patient.)

If earache occurs in the middle of the night, conservative measures may be safely instituted at home until the child is examined by his physician the following day. Some practical suggestions for the relief of pain are the use of ear drops such as auralgan which requires a prescription, or warm sweet oil inserted in the ear every four hours. Be sure the patient lies on his opposite side for ten minutes to allow the ear drops to run deep enough to be of value. Resting the ear on a hot water bottle or a heating pad turned on low works wonders. A teaspoon of baby's cough syrup, particularly if it contains codeine, provides great relief. Remember that aspirin with tempra or tylenol are used for the relief of pain— not only for fever.

All suspected cases of otitis media should be seen by your physician. The specific treatment of ear infection consists of:

1. Nose drops which shrink the mucous membrane of the nose and thus help keep the eustachian tube free of obstruction.
2. Antihistamines to help dry up the mucous.
3. Antibiotic to eradicate the organism causing the infection.

Treatment should be continued for a minimum of seven to ten days and not just until the patient feels better. This allows fluid or pus behind the ear drum to be completely absorbed. Until this happens hearing loss may be present. Normal hearing will completely return, however, when the infection is cured with appropriate therapy.

The commonest cause of hearing loss in children is an inadequate response to the therapy of otitis media. Therefore, no matter how well the child may be responding to treatment in your opinion, it is mandatory that the ears be rechecked.

Occasionally, the ear drum (tympanic membrane) ruptures spontaneously. This occurs when the pressure behind it builds up from entrapped fluid or pus. Fortunately, a ruptured ear drum usually heals promptly within a few days. If the ear drum is bulging when examined by your doctor, a myringotomy may be necessary. This is a surgical incision in the ear drum which allows for proper drainage of the entrapped fluid or pus. With sedation this may be easily accomplished in the doctor's office. Such an incision will heal promptly.

Mastoiditis used to be a common complication of otitis media before the advent of antibiotic therapy. It is an infection of the bone in the back of the ear. The diagnosis is suspected when pressure on this area causes acute pain and is confirmed by X ray. Surgical drainage is often necessary.

B. External Otitis. In this condition the ear canal which extends inward from the outside of the ear to the ear drum (tympanic membrane) becomes red and swollen. It is similar to an infected scratch. Do not confuse it with a middle ear infection which is behind the ear drum. The chief complaint is ear pain. External otitis is usually bacterial in origin. Treatment consists of ear drops containing antibiotics and a pain killer. Some practical points for the relief of ear pain were discussed under otitis media. All suspected cases should be seen by your physician. He is the only one capable of distinguishing this from otitis media and other types of external otitis.

C. Swimmer's Ear (Fungus). Swimmer's ear is an external otitis caused by a fungus. The major symptom is severe ear pain. Pulling on the ear lobe increases the pain. Treatment consists of alleviating the pain with antifungal ear drops and preventing additional water from getting into the external ear canal. Aspirin in the recommended dosage will often not be strong enough to relieve the pain. Therefore, codeine may be prescribed by your physician. Swimming must be forbidden until the child is well and if he showers he must wear a bathing cap. Treatment should be continued for a minimum of a week even if the signs and symptoms disappear sooner to prevent a rapid recurrence.

It is possible to prevent many cases of swimmer's ear by using alcohol routinely after swimming. Place two drops in each ear. Alcohol evaporates rapidly and thus dries the ear canal. Ear plugs are not satisfactory. All cases should be seen by your physician. He is the only one capable of distinguishing this type of external otitis from other types and from otitis media.

EAR WAX

Ear wax will often drain by itself, a little bit at a time. Mother will notice some on the infant's sheet. This is normal. If mother is having a difficult time keeping the external ear canal clean because of a great deal of wax, try Debrox. Debrox is available in the drugstore without a prescription. Squeeze five drops into each ear twice daily for three days. Then remove the softened wax by gently cleaning with warm water.

EATING HABITS—UNDERWEIGHT

Most thin children are perfectly healthy. I think the real problem with thinness is what the parents are afraid of. A complete checkup will detect any disease condition. Given time, a child free of disease will gain weight. The child with an eating problem is no more susceptible to illnesses than any other child, and no child has ever

136

starved to death regulating his own diet. With additives to most foods we eat, it is almost impossible to develop nutritional deficiencies. Some children will eat a great deal and not gain weight, others will eat very little and gain weight. The individual appetite varies.

Meals should be made as pleasant as possible. If your child likes only a few foods, accept it. There is no need for a wide variety of the same types of foods. Do not force the child to taste any food that he really dislikes or use the threat of no dessert. The food which is refused at a previous meal should not be re-served.

Generally, it is best to serve less than the child will eat. Small feedings do not make a child small. Let the child ask for more if he wants it. The average child will be able to feed himself between twelve and eighteen months of age. If mother shows a great deal of hostility or anxiety, it is probably best that she not be in the room when the child is eating. The child should not be bribed to eat all of his food. Do not say all the poor people in the world would like his food. One answer I heard was "give it to the poor." Parents must accept the fact that children love to eat hamburgers, hot dogs, and drink Coke. These foods are not harmful. Given a choice of going to a restaurant where the child may sit down at the table and be served roast beef or steak, the child would much rather go to the local hamburger haven.

Some children cannot eat enough to gain weight because they are tense and nervous. This uses up extra energy. Don't try to push the child into eating more. Being thin may be a family characteristic. Many individual differences in body size and proportions are built up through growth processes controlled by heredity and environment. Extra rest is not helpful if the child has already grown out of the routine. There are many preparations on the market which supposedly will increase the appetite. Occasionally, one of these appetite stimulants will work for a brief period of time. My favorite preparation is Zentron Chewable Tablets, which are available in the drugstore without a prescription. Take one tablet twice a day. However, I do not believe it is helpful to give an appetite stimulant for more than thirty days.

Children who become thin because of an acute illness will regain their weight rapidly when they are well.

ECZEMA (ATOPIC DERMATITIS)

Eczema is a very troublesome skin disease of infancy and child-hood. Thirty per cent of the cases begin at or before three months of age and continue throughout the first two years of life. Eczema between the ages of two and six years is rare, and after six years of age extremely rare.

Eczema is an allergic response on the part of the individual patient to something he is sensitive to. It is characterized by flat, raised, red lesions or lesions with a small amount of fluid called vesicles. The little vesicles may coalesce and rupture causing serum to be expelled onto the surface of the skin. Crusting is common when the serum dries. Often there is scaling and at times accentuation of the normal skin markings. Itching is almost always present. There is a high incidence of secondary infection. Eczema is commonly located behind the ears and knees and in front of the elbow joints. If it becomes chronic, there may be increased pigmentation (coloring) of the skin. Eczema is notorious for spontaneous remissions and exacerbations. It often clears spontaneously in the presence of acute febrile infections. Often the eruption of teeth causes eczema to become worse.

Treatment consists of compressing the affected areas for thirty minutes three times a day with normal saline or Burrow's solution. Normal saline solution, acceptable for this purpose, can readily be made by adding one level teaspoonful of table salt to one pint of water. Burrow's solution may be made by dissolving one Domeboro Powder in a quart of water. Domeboro Powders are available in the drugstore without a prescription. Calamine (Caladryl) lotion may be used to minimize scratching. It is available in the drugstore without a prescription. Antihistamines are valuable in reducing the itching. (See Colds.) Keep finger nails cut short. Cortisone ointments are available, which are not absorbed from the skin and often provide a dramatic temporary cure. Occasionally, cortisone may have to be given orally or by injection. Hypoallergenic soaps such as Lowila Cake that do not irritate the skin are useful. It is available in the drugstore without a prescription. Hypoallergic formulas may be helpful. (See Formulas—Prosobee.) It should be emphasized that changing from whole milk to evaporated milk to skim milk or Similac is of no value, as basically these

138

products are prepared from cow's milk. A diet free from wheat, eggs, milk, and citrus may be of value. The manufacturers of different baby foods have supplied your physician with a list of their foods which are free from these products. However, these manufacturers' lists cannot be used interchangeably since the base of their foods may be different. Antibiotic therapy is necessary for secondary infection.

In resistant cases or those cases in which chronic skin changes are occurring, skin testing is in order. A vaccine is then made up based upon the test results and hypodesensitization shots given. (See Allergy and The Allergic Patient.) It is hard to evaluate the treatment of eczema because the natural course of the illness is exacerbations and recovery regardless of therapy. Control and prevention of chronic skin changes should be the goal. If a child has one major manifestation of allergy, such as eczema, he is more apt to develop other major manifestations of allergy, which include perennial allergic rhinitis and asthma. (See Allergic Nose, Asthma.)

EMPHYSEMA (CHRONIC LUNG DISEASE)

If a mucous plug obstructs the small bronchi which carries air to the lungs, the part furthest from the obstruction will become distended. This distention of the sac-like structures of the lungs where air is exchanged is called emphysema. Emphysema develops over a long period of time. Consequently, its victims are frequently not aware of the fact that their lung capacity is being slowly nibbled away, until one day they are stunned to realize that they tire easily, run out of breath after slight exertion, and that their nagging cough has never gone away. A patient described it as someone constantly holding a pillow over his face. You try to take a full breath of air but you never can. Emphysema is now recognized as a national epidemic in the United States.

The signs and symptoms of emphysema are:

1. Shortness of breath.
2. Blueness of the lips.
3. Difficulty in breathing when lying down.
4. A barrelled chest.
5. Persistent cough.
6. Weight loss.

Emphysema is a sign of chronic lung disease. The primary causes are polluted air, chronic lung infections, and cigarette smoking. It is often secondary to asthma. (See Asthma.) Emphysema is not a common problem in children because it takes a long time to develop. However, if emphysema is to be prevented in the adult, children must have vigorous treatment of all disease conditions that may cause it.

The best treatment of emphysema is prevention. Once emphysema has developed, it is not reversible. A person with emphysema may have to curtail many normal activities. It is most important for a patient with emphysema to get a flu shot every year to help prevent complications of the flu, such as pneumonia. (See Immunizations.)

ENCEPHALITIS

Encephalitis means that the brain is inflamed (infected).

The signs and symptoms of encephalitis may be sudden or gradual in their appearance. They consist of:

1. Drowsiness.
2. Hyperactivity.
3. Irritability.
4. Twitchings.
5. Convulsions.
6. Coma.
7. Loss of muscle power.
8. Speech disturbances.
9. Difficulty in walking.
10. Abnormal reflexes.

Encephalitis may occur as a complication of some of the usual childhood illnesses such as measles and chicken pox, or as a primary disease, usually due to a virus. Certain types of encephalitis may be spread by the mosquito or other arthropods. An arthropod is any segmented invertebrate having jointed legs. The mosquito carries the virus of encephalitis after biting an animal which acts as a reservoir for the virus.

The diagnosis is confirmed by performing a lumbar puncture (spinal tap). The spinal fluid obtained is analyzed for certain specific changes that occur. (See Spinal Tap.)

Treatment consists of general supportive measures which include adequate fluid balance, rest, and prevention of anemia. No specific antibiotic is of value since encephalitis is a viral infection.

Complications are pronounced mental and emotional changes which may appear even after the acute phase is over. Some cases are more serious than others. The patient usually recovers, but the outlook is always guarded as to any pronounced mental and emotional changes.

ENEMAS

Since enemas are potentially dangerous for young children they should not be given by the parents. Plain water enemas may lead to water intoxication, since water may be absorbed from the intestine. If the child is complaining of abdominal pain or vomiting, an enema should never be given. Under these circumstances there is always the possibility of a surgical condition of the abdomen such as appendicitis, and an enema could rupture the intestine.

Enemas may be given to older children by their parents on the advice of their doctor. Enemas are useful in preparing the child for X-ray examinations of the abdomen and in the treatment of some cases of worms following medication. Fleet's enemas are available in disposable plastic containers at the drugstore without a prescription. These are much easier to use than the old-fashioned enema bag. Be sure to ask your pharmacist for the pediatric size.

EPIGLOTTITIS

When a child opens his mouth and depresses his tongue, the little round swelling seen in the back of the throat is called the epiglottis. Inflammation of this structure is called epiglottitis. This infection may occur at any age, but is most frequent in young children.

A. Signs and Symptoms.   The signs and symptoms of epiglottitis are similiar to croup. The child becomes suddenly ill. There is a loud barking noise. The patient has difficulty in getting air in. The throat is sore. Fever may or may not be present. There is usually little or no hoarseness. Respiratory distress may develop rapidly. The signs and symptoms of respiratory distress are sucking in, in the neck, between the ribs, under the rib cage, and moving in and out of the nose as the child breathes

141

B. Etiology (Cause).   Most cases are believed to be caused by a specific bacteria.

C. Treatment.   This disease is considered a pediatric emergency. The airway can become completely closed off as the epiglottis becomes markedly swollen. All cases should be hospitalized. The principles of therapy are outlined under Croup: oxygen, humidity, antibiotic, steroid, and careful observation. Most children respond dramatically to treatment. Should the patient fail to improve or if blueness occurs and persists, a tracheotomy may have to be performed. (See Croup.)

ERYTHREMA MULTIFORME

Erythrema multiforme is an allergic reaction. It consists of giant hives which vary in size and shape almost hourly. This condition is not serious however frightening the rash may look. The exact cause is unknown, but infection may be a precipitating factor. Adrenalin, cortisone and antihistamines are your physician's weapons to counteract this condition. Any underlying infection must be adequately treated. Caladryl lotion (calamine) may be used to control itching if necessary. It is available in the drugstore without a prescription. Even with treatment the rash usually remains for a few days. There are occasional recurrences.

ERYTHROBLASTOSIS—HEMOLYTIC
(DISEASE OF THE NEWBORN)

In order for erythroblastosis to develop it is necessary for the mother to lack a blood factor that the fetus possesses. Erythroblastosis develops in the following way: An RH positive man marries an RH negative woman and they conceive an RH positive baby. The RH positive factor of the baby's blood gains access into the circulatory system of the mother by the passage of RH positive fetal red blood cells across the placental barrier into the mother's circulation, or accidentally by a previous RH positive blood transfusion. The mother produces antibodies against the fetal RH positive red blood cells and these antibodies enter the fetal circulation causing destruction of the fetal red blood cells.

Statistics indicate that twelve out of one hundred marriages in the United States are between RH negative women and RH positive men. However, only one in two hundred pregnancies result in an infant affected with erythroblastosis. It is rare for this condition to occur in the first born child, even when the proper blood setup is present, but the probability of an affected infant increases with each successive pregnancy when the baby is RH positive.

The signs and symptoms of erythroblastosis are:

1. Anemia due to the rapid destruction of the fetal red blood cells.
2. Jaundice (yellowness). One of the breakdown products of the baby's red blood cells is bilirubin. The newborn baby has a limited capacity to metabolize (handle) bilirubin causing the infant to become jaundiced.
3. Edema (swelling), particularly of the hands and feet.
4. Enlargement of the liver.
5. Enlargement of the spleen.

To compensate for the anemia new red cells are rapidly produced by the baby. Many of these new red cells are still not fully developed and are called erythroblasts; thus, the name of the disease.

Anemia, if severe, will impair heart function and lead to heart failure, which in turn leads to the accumulation of fluid (edema). Brain damage, known as kernicterus, is the most serious complication of erythroblastosis. *Brain damage results from the accumulation of high levels of bilirubin within the first five days of life. A bilirubin concentration greater than 20 milligrams per cent statistically increases the chance of brain damage so that vigorous treatment is indicated to prevent it.*

Good obstetrical management is very important in the early anticipation and recognition of a baby affected with erythroblastosis. A careful history must be obtained regarding all previous labors and deliveries. All pregnant women must have routine blood typing, including RH determination, and if the expectant mother is RH negative, her husband should also have his blood typed. All RH negative women should also be followed by serial determinations of antibodies to the RH factor. A rising titer may indicate a fetus affected by the disease.

The baby's physician is already alerted to the possibility of erythroblastosis occurring by adequate prenatal testing by your

143

obstetrician. At birth the infant's RH type is determined and other blood tests are done to determine his condition.

An exciting discovery has recently shown that light from 10 twenty-watt daylight bulbs is a safe and effective method of preventing bilirubin build-up. This prophylactic approach may be all that is necessary in very mild cases. In other mild cases the only treatment necessary may be repeated single blood transfusions to correct the anemia. In severe cases one or more exchange transfusions are necessary. In order to determine the proper treatment, your physician will carefully follow the level of your baby's bilirubin and perform other laboratory tests. The physician's most important job is to prevent brain damage. The risk of brain damage is almost eliminated if the bilirubin is kept below 20 miligrams per cent, but treatment must take place before brain damage occurs. Once brain damage has occurred it is not reversible. An exchange transfusion lowers the baby's bilirubin. It is performed by inserting a plastic catheter into the umbilical vein and then alternately withdrawing and introducing small amounts of blood. This is considered a major operative procedure. An exchange transfusion of 500 cc's of fresh whole blood will remove approximately eighty-five per cent of the infant's original blood, thereby removing many of the sensitized cells, and thus reducing the degree of red blood cell destruction. This prevents a further rise in bilirubin. In selected cases the early induction of labor may be necessary, although this carries with it the increased risk and hazards of prematurity (see prematurity).

The outlook for all RH positive infants of sensitized mothers is good. With experience, early detection and treatment, the mortality of live born babies with erythroblastosis is usually between four and eight per cent. However, once a mother has delivered a stillborn, caused by erythroblastosis, most of her subsequent RH positive babies will also be stillborn.

Since the major problem before birth is one of anemia, modern medicine has now developed a technique by which the baby may be given a blood transfusion while still in utero. That is, the baby may be given a transfusion prior to birth.

A most dramatic breakthrough in the treatment of this disease was made in 1967, which will change the entire problem. *This disease now appears to be preventable* by the use of a special low dose of anti-RH gamma globulin. This has proved effective in the prevention of RH sensitization in RH negative mothers. This suggests that a prophylactic program may be initiated for all unsensitized RH negative mothers. This low dose of anti-RH gamma globulin is given intramuscularly within seventy-two hours of delivery in the prevention of RH sensitization. However, treatment of this disease will still be necessary until this program or some other program is in wide use, to prevent erythroblastosis.

EYES

A. Astigmatism. This is a condition of the eye in which parallel rays of light from an external source converge and diverge unequally in different meridians. The meridian of the eye is a line passing around the eyeball.

B. Boric Acid. I do not like to recommend boric acid solutions for the eyes because if a mistake is made in its preparation, the eyes may be injured. If the parents desire to use boric acid, I would suggest getting it from your druggist and telling him what it is for so that he can be doubly sure that it is not too strong.

C. Color Blindness. Color blindness is the inability to recognize red, green, blue, or some combination of these colors. Usually the child lacks perception in varying degrees for one or two colors. It is hereditary in nature, but the exact cause is not known. It occurs ten times more frequently in males than in females. While it is incurable, color sense can be developed to some extent. Color blind people readily learn to recognize traffic signals as uniformly the red stop light is the top light and green is the bottom light. Such a child, however, may need help in the choice of clothes to avoid color combinations that do not blend well, but that is not a very serious problem.

D. Crossed Eyes (Strabismus, Squint, Lazy Eyes). Strabismus is a disorder of vision due to the turning of one or both eyes from their normal position, so that both cannot be directed at the same point together. A transient deviation of the eyes during the first months of life is seldom significant as it usually disappears without treatment. Any persistent deviation should be investigated. The longer the child's eyes remain in a misaligned state, the greater the chances for abnormal vision. Children can develop blindness from improper use of an eye. There is little reason for children to

145

develop permanent eye trouble when the condition is diagnosed early enough, and watched carefully. Remember those well-baby visits during the first year of life, and routine check-ups thereafter.

A crossed eye is treated by patching the good eye. This forces the bad eye to work in an effort to correct the muscle imbalance. Improvement is often dramatic, thus avoiding the necessity of eye surgery. Even if surgery is eventually necessary, the results are excellent. If a refractive error is present, glasses are prescribed. In children under twelve months of age, eye drops are used instead of glasses.

E. Eye Tests.   Although trained volunteers can accurately test the vision in youngsters three or four years of age, thus preventing many cases of blindness, there is some under referral no matter what system is used. For example, it is entirely possible for a child to read standard E charts accurately and have a severe disturbance in vision. All children should have a routine eye examination by a qualified specialist prior to starting school, or sooner if the parents are suspicious about the possibility of any eye problem. A qualified specialist is an ophthalmologist, that is a doctor who specializes in diseases of the eye. An optometrist, although he examines eyes, is not a qualified specialist. He does not have a medical degree and by law is prevented from using certain medications which are useful in the proper examination of the eye. His primary responsibility is that of filling prescriptions for glasses.

F. Farsightedness.   Presbyopia is another term. A farsighted person cannot see things near him. This condition is correctable with glasses.

G. Foreign Body—Corneal Ulceration.   A foreign body in the eye may scratch the cornea. The cornea is the transparent part of the external coat of the eye that covers the colored portion. If there is a question of irritation of the eye or a questionable history of a foreign body, the child should be seen by his physician. The history must be carefully checked. Can the parent be sure that only sand got in the eyes? Is there a possibility of a mixture of sand and lime from a construction site down the street? Corneal ulcerations cannot be seen with the naked eye. Your physician will therefore stain the eye with a harmless dye called fluorscein, which will turn any corneal ulcerations green. A corneal ulceration is treated with antibiotic eye drops. An eye patch is placed over the affected eye.

146

This condition is followed closely to make sure that complete healing occurs. This usually takes place in forty-eight to seventy-two hours, depending on the depth of the ulceration. With deep ulcerations pain is present. Aspirin may be given. If a corneal ulceration does not heal promptly without infection, scar tissue may result that can interfere with vision.

H. Glasses. (1) *Safety Lenses.* Eye glasses for children should be made with safety lenses that will not break. (2) *Contact Lenses.* Contact lenses have been developed which are perfectly safe to wear and do not injure the eye. Most people cannot wear them, however, for more than ten to twelve hours per day. Tolerance to contact lenses must be gradually built up. Psychologically, contact lenses are good for the individual.

I. Nearsightedness. Myopia is another term. A nearsighted person cannot see things far away. It is the commonest eye problem that occurs in children. Myopia occurs most frequently after six years of age and can be of fairly sudden onset. The teacher may notice that the child is having trouble reading the blackboard at school or is holding his book closer than usual. This condition is correctable with glasses.

J. Pink Eye (Conjunctivitis). Pink eye is an inflammation of the inner aspect of the eyelids. A pussy discharge is usually found in the corner of the eyes. In severe cases the eyelids may be stuck together and swollen. Pink eye is usually a bacterial or viral infection. Some cases may be allergic in origin. Many cases are self-limited and need no specific treatment. For mild cases Visine Eye Drops are available in the drugstore without a prescription. Use one or two drops in each eye four times a day. Both eyes should be treated even if only one eye is involved since the infection spreads easily. If the child fails to respond in a day or two, your physician should be consulted. Permanent eye damage is almost unheard of. Be sure, however, that medication put in the eye is specially prepared for that purpose. All other medications may cause serious damage. Solutions made for the eyes are called ophthalmic. Do not confuse this with ear solutions referred to as otic. A few preparations are made for combined use in the eyes and ears.

Pink eye is very common in the newborn since the infant recently passed through mother's birth canal, which like all parts of the body contains many bacteria. Routinely, silver nitrate drops or

147

some kind of antibiotic preparation is placed in the baby's eyes after delivery as a preventive measure. Most physicians feel silver nitrate has proved to be somewhat irritating. Therefore, antibiotic eye preparations are preferred.

K. Sties. A sty is an infection in the hair follicle of the eyelid. It may come to a head and break spontaneously. The use of warm soaks for at least twenty minutes four times a day is helpful. Antibiotic eye ointment may be necessary. Sties are difficult to cure because when they rupture the infection easily spreads to other hair follicles. If a sty is getting progressively worse, your physician should be consulted.

L. Tearing—Obstruction of the Nasolacrimal Duct. The nasolacrimal duct handles the discharge of tears and normal secretion from the eyes. If the duct is obstructed at birth, tearing occurs from the involved eye. Usually only one eye is involved. Massage a few times a day may re-establish proper drainage. Start with gentle pressure at the inside corner of the eye, work slightly towards the bridge of the nose and then down along the side of the nose. If in doubt, ask your physician to show you how it is done. Repeat this procedure for five minutes every day. If massage does not reestablish proper drainage within a month or two, this duct may have to be opened by probing it, generally under anesthesia. This nearly always works. The cure is usually permanent.

F

FEEDING—WHEN, WHAT AND HOW TO (ALSO SEE FORMULAS AND VITAMINS)

A. Schedule vs. Demand Feeding. All babies are individuals and no strict schedule should be forced down their throats. Most babies will adjust to every four hour feedings quite nicely. Some small infants may need to be fed every three hours. Others may want to sleep for five or six hours at a time.

Demand feeding means that the baby is fed whenever he wants to be. However, this does not seem practical during the middle of supper while the rest of the family waits. The main consideration is that the baby does not go hungry for any long period of time. Having the baby wait a half hour is not going to hurt anybody. Try to reach a happy medium between schedule and demand feeding.

B. Feeding Every Four Hours.   Six a.m., ten a.m., two p.m., six p.m., ten p.m., two a.m. There is nothing magic in this schedule which seems to be universal. Be flexible and change the hours if it is more convenient by starting at 7, 8 or 9 a.m.

C. Feeding—Every Two Hours.   No baby at home needs to be fed every two hours. Do not be misled by the sucking reflex or by an over-active baby. Food is not necessary every time an infant cries. The baby's stomach needs rest too.

D. Feeding with a Bottle Holder.   Babies should not be fed with a bottle holder. Milk can be aspirated into their lungs which may cause pneumonia. With a bottle holder it is impossible to keep the neck of the bottle filled to prevent the swallowing of additional air which may lead to colic. Hold the baby while feeding him. The closeness that develops with the parents during this time is important.

E. Skipping the Two a.m. Feeding.   Most infants will give up the two a.m. feeding when they weigh approximately twelve pounds.

F. Water.   Many newborn babies will not drink water between feedings. If this is the case, no harm will be done.

G. Sugar Water.   It is not necessary to add sugar to the baby's water, but if he prefers it that way the suggested amount is one level tablespoon for each pint of water.

H. Well Water.   Before giving well water to the baby, have it tested by the State Health Department. This service is provided free of charge. A bacteria count tells us if the water is safe to drink. Well water should also be tested for nitrate salts. Nitrate salts can cause blueness of the lips and skin by combining with the infant's blood, thus interfering with oxygen exchange.

I. Formulas, Amount Taken.   Newborn babies, especially in the first week of life, drink very little formula. The average amount taken at a feeding is about one half to one ounce. They are slow, pokey eaters. By two to four weeks of age, the infant will probably take five ounces at each feeding. Forcing the baby to take so many ounces at each feeding attempts to make the baby a machine, which he is not. Only the baby knows whether he is hungry or not.

149

He does not understand nutrition and minor variations in formulas.
This is only important to the scientist and nutritionist.

J. Formula—Increase. If the baby is eagerly taking three
ounces of formula in each bottle every four hours, and continues to
act hungry, increase the amount offered to four and one-half or five
ounces. I always like to see the baby leave a little bit of formula
in the bottle. Then I know he is getting enough. The total amount
of formula given during a twenty-four hour period should not exceed thirty-two ounces at any age. Milk is deficient in iron. It is
far from the perfect food. Additional caloric requirements should
come from solid foods. (See Anemia—Iron Deficiency.)

K. Evaporated Milk—How Long to Give It. Undiluted
evaporated milk is twice the strength of whole milk. When evaporated milk is diluted with an equal amount of water, it is similar
to whole milk and may be used indefinitely. The last time I counted
there were forty-two brands of evaporated milk sold under four
hundred and sixty different names. The chief reason for the widespread use of whole milk is that it tastes better to most people.

L. Solids—When to Start. Solids are generally started at
about one month of age. Babies who receive solids at this time seem
to be more contented and are inclined to relinquish the two a.m.
feeding sooner. There is some evidence in the literature that starting
solids too early is harmful because the infant cannot handle the
additional sodium intake. Solids seem to satisfy most infants' ap-
petites for a longer period of time than their formula. A suggested
schedule for starting solids is:

> (a) One month of age—cereal. Rice cereal, because it is almost
> universally tolerated, is the first solid food started—one or two
> teaspoons (dry measure) in the morning and evening. Mix the
> cereal with the formula so it is like a thick soup and give it on a
> spoon. Gradually increase the amount given to up to four table-
> spoons twice a day as your baby's appetite increases. At times a
> baby will refuse; do not force him.
>
> (b) Two months of age—fruit. Applesauce and banana are
> recommended for the baby's first fruits, as these are the least
> allergenic. Start with one or two teaspoons at noon and offer more
> —up to one jar—as the baby's appetite increases. Fruits, particu-
> larly prunes, may cause the infant's stools to become loose. If this
> occurs, reduce the amount of this particular fruit or avoid it.

150

(c) Three months of age—vegetables and egg yolk. Yellow vegetables are recommended first. Then introduce the green vegetables, and alternate them by the jar. Start with one or two teaspoons at noon and as the baby's appetite increases offer more— up to one jar a day. Spinach is a good source of iron, but most babies dislike it. Accept the baby's wishes. Spinach may cause the baby to have loose stools. If this occurs, avoid it or decrease the amount given. Egg yolk may be started by three months of age. It comes already prepared, or you may hard boil an egg yourself. Egg yolk is a good food because it is an important source of iron. Avoid egg white (albumin) until the child is a year of age as it is an important cause of food allergy. Thus, scrambled or soft cooked eggs are not given before a year of age.

(d) Four months of age—meat. Lamb, chicken and beef are recommended for the baby's first meats. Start with one or two teaspoons in the evening and as the baby's appetite increases offer more—up to one jar. Pork is best avoided until one year of age, as it is harder to digest. Liver is an excellent source of iron, but most babies dislike it. I suggest offering liver, but not forcing it down the baby's throat. Fish may be substituted for meat.

(e) Six months of age—all the fancy foods including baby soups and desserts. Juice is usually offered between feedings at any age if the baby is hungry. Orange juice was generally given before the advent of multivitamin drops because of its vitamin C content, but it is no longer essential. Many babies are allergic to orange juice or are constantly spitting it up; therefore, I do not recommend it. Apple juice seems to be more universally tolerated. I do not recommend prepared baby juices as they are quite expensive. Use regular juice diluted with an equal amount of water. Cod liver oil is no longer necessary in any baby's diet.

FISH HOOK

Do not pull on a fish hook. A bob is present that will rip the skin. The hook is pushed forward through the skin after cutting part of it off with pliers. This minimizes further tissue damage. The wound is then thoroughly soaked in Phisohex. A tetanus booster is given when the date of the last immunization is more than one year ago. The signs and symptoms of secondary infection must be carefully watched for—heat, tenderness, pain and swelling—if they occur consult your physician again.

FLAT FEET

If your baby's foot looks flat, it is. The normal foot of an infant is fatter and wider than that of an adult. It seldom has a longitudinal arch and never a transverse one. Instead, babies have fat pads. As they grow the pads gradually disappear and an arch becomes apparent.

Even if the feet remain flat, they are perfectly normal functioning feet. Unfortunately, for cultural reasons, flat feet carry a certain stigma in the United States which is ridiculous. As a matter of fact, a flat foot is a better functioning foot than one which has an extremely high arch where the weight is not evenly distributed. Corrective shoes are not necessary for flat feet, in my opinion. No physician can create a new arch. However, the attitude of the physician towards flat feet will vary a great deal, depending upon his training. Some physicians will honestly prescribe corrective shoes. Occasionally, this is due to pressures brought to bear on the doctor by the parents. How, then, can we explain the difference in recommendations between the same type of specialists regarding this problem? The explanation is simply this: If any improvement takes place with corrective shoes, the physician who prescribed them gives credit to the shoe. The physician who does not prescribe corrective shoes gives credit for any improvement to normal growth and development.

FOOD POISONING—SALMONELLA INFECTIONS

Salmonellosis is increasing at an alarming rate in the United States. It seems to be increasing because the bacteria salmonella can be harbored by almost any animal, domestic or wild. Salmonella organisms have been found in not only almost any kind of domestic livestock and poultry, but even in fish, snakes, lizards, turtles and insects. "Typhoid Mary" the story of yesteryear has been replaced by a new innocent carrier of disease "Salmonella Sam." The Food and Drug Administration estimates that among every ten thousand people, twenty-five may be unsuspected carriers of the organism. The carrier is free of symptoms, but may contaminate all he touches. If parents are suspicious that recently ingested food was spoiled there is no reason to call your physician immediately as nothing can

152

be done to prevent the child from becoming sick. Pumping out the stomach is of no value as the bacteria are not washed out.

The signs and symptoms are acute onset of vomiting and diarrhea which is usually accompanied by fever, headache and nausea. Abdominal cramping often occurs. Sometimes there is blood and mucous in the stool. There are many different types of salmonella organisms that produce food poisoning. The mode of transmission is by water, milk and food which has become contaminated by carriers, and indirectly by flies. The incubation period is six hours to seven days. Numerous antibiotics are effective against salmonella infections. (See Typhoid.)

FORMULAS

There is no doubt that ninety-five per cent or more of all babies can take any milk formula. All but special formulas are composed of milk. There is no basic difference between any kind of evaporated milk on the market nor between whole milk and evaporated milk. The source of all milk is the cow. If you use evaporated milk, buy the least expensive brand. Many parents are prone to change formulas for any reason whatsoever, and then announce that the child's problem is solved. I seriously doubt that the change cured the problem. There is no medical rationale for this type of thinking. If a special formula is recommended by your physician, it should be tried for at least one week. This amount of time is required for the previous formula to be completely eliminated from the infant's system.

Are formulas really necessary? Yes, they are. The use of whole milk at birth, even though it may be tolerated, places too great a load on the newborn's kidneys. It is like driving a new car at high speed.

Formulas are kept in the refrigerator to inhibit the growth of bacteria. Prepare only two days' supply at a time. Scientific studies have proven that the baby will thrive equally well whether the formula is given cold, at room temperature, or warmed. Follow your baby's personal preference.

The instructions given below for the preparation of various formulas include the use of water. Sterilize this water or use the terminal method of formula preparation.

1. Evaporated Milk Formulas. An evaporated milk formula which is suitable for the vast majority of babies consists of thirteen ounces of evaporated milk, seventeen ounces of water and two tablespoons of some type of sugar, such as Dextri-Maltose 1, or Karo. The sugar is added to provide enough calories for adequate growth and development.

2. Prepared Formulas—Similac, Enfamil, etc. The most popular prepared formulas are Similac and Enfamil. Other prepared formulas include: Bakers Modified Milk, Bremil, Carnalac, Formil, Lactum, Modilac, Optimil, and S.M.A. In spite of claims by the manufacturers, there is no significant difference among them that affects your baby's growth and development. Ask your doctor which one he prefers.

Some type of sugar is added to a prepared formula by the manufacturer. They are sold as a liquid or powder, and are ready for use when mixed with water. The liquid is generally found in a 13-ounce can. Mix one can of liquid with one can of water, and divide the total amount into the number of bottles needed in twenty-four hours.

Each can of powdered formula contains a measuring spoon. Add one measure of powder to each 2 ounces of water. For example, 6 ounces of formula is made by adding three measures of the powder to 6 ounces of water. Sometimes it is difficult to get the powder to mix well with water; therefore, most mothers prefer the liquid.

An additional advantage of prepared formulas is that they contain all the necessary vitamins and minerals, thus eliminating the need for additional vitamins which are frequently forgotten or spit up. In my opinion babies on prepared formulas gain weight faster and have less colic than those on evaporated milk.

Similac and Enfamil are also available with iron. Additional iron is not routinely needed. However, formulas with iron are particularly useful in the premature infant where iron stores are deficient and in the prevention of anemia in children who do not eat enough meat. The preparation of formulas with iron is the same as those without iron.

3. Ready-to-Use Formulas. Ready-to-use formulas in a throwaway bottle with a disposable nipple may be purchased in most drugstores. They contain all the necessary vitamins and minerals. For test purposes they have been stored without refrigeration for over a year and have remained sterile. Ready-to-use formulas are a convenience that cost more but make vacations more pleasant. Keep a few bottles around the house for emergency situations.

4. Lactic Acid Formulas. Lactic acid formulas are sold under various trade names in different parts of the country. They are prepared from cow's milk by adding various healthful bacteria to the milk to modify it. This type of formula is ready for use as purchased in the grocery store. Home delivery is frequently available.

When travelling away from your usual source, capsules may be obtained that can be added to whole milk which produce the same results.

This type of formula is most helpful as an intermediary in switching your baby from a soybean preparation prior to the introduction of whole milk. Wonders are often worked in persistent cases of diarrhea.

5. Soybean Formulas (Prosobee, Sobee, Soyalac, Isomil, Neo-mull-soy, and Mulsoy. These formulas are prepared from the soybean. Their differences are only important to the nutritionist. Soybean formulas are used as milk substitutes. Research indicates that they may be helpful in delaying the development of allergies. Thus, if a newborn has extremely allergic parents or siblings, it may be worthwhile to keep him off milk during the first year of life.

Soybean formulas have a characteristic smell and cause the stools to be slightly loose. Prosobee, Isomil and Neo-mull-soy will provide a product that looks similar to regular milk. The others look brown. All these products are available in liquid form. Standard dilution is one can of liquid to one can of water. Mulsoy, Sobee and Soyalac are also available in a powdered form. Standard dilution is one tablespoon to each two ounces of water. Measuring scoops equivalent to one tablespoon are usually provided in the can. To make larger amounts one level 8-ounce measuring cup of powdered formula may be added to one quart of water.

6. Probana. This is a therapeutic formula suitable for feeding infants and children with the celiac syndrome, or malabsorption due to various causes. It is sometimes used when a patient is re-

155

covering from diarrhea. It is supplied in a powder only. Normal dilution is one measure found inside the can to 2 ounces of water. (See Celiac Disease.)

7. Meat Base Formulas (Beef and Lamb).   Meat base formulas are for children who are allergic to milk or soybeans. They are prepared from strained beef and strained lamb. The standard dilution for the beef base formula is one can of liquid to one and one-half to two cans of water, depending upon the child's age. The standard dilution for the lamb base formula is one can of liquid to one can of water.

8. Nutramigen.   This formula contains predigested protein; thus, some of the work in the digestive tract has already been done in the laboratory. Nutramigen is ideal for some allergic infants and is necessary for those that may have an inborn error of metabolism such as occurs in galactosemia. Galactosemia is a very rare condition characterized by inability to convert sugar in a normal fashion. Nutramigen comes in a powder only. Each can contains a measuring spoon. Add one measure of powder to each 2 ounces of water, or one level 8-ounce measuring cup to a quart of water.

9. Lofenalac.   (See Phenylketonuria.)

10. Olac, Alacta.   These formulas are high in protein. Many physicians use them to feed premature infants. Olac is supplied in a liquid and powder. Alacta is supplied as a powder only. The liquid is mixed with an equal amount of water, and the powder is mixed by adding a packed level measure found inside the can to 2 ounces of water, or one level 8-ounce measuring cup to one quart of water.

11. Similac PM-60-40.   This formula is used for those infants who would benefit from lowered mineral and protein levels, or for those infants who are predisposed to developing a low level of blood calcium. Similac PM-60-40 is supplied in cans containing one pound of powder. One measure (found inside the can) is mixed with 2 ounces of water.

12. Cho-free.   This formula is used when selected sugars are indicated as in recurrent diarrhea associated with the loss of specific sugars such as lactose and sucrose. It may also be used as a milk substitute in the dietary management of galactosemia. The caloric value is adjusted by the regulation of the type and amount of carbohydrates used when the formula is reconstituted. Cho-free is prepared by placing 13 ounces of water into a clean saucepan and adding the desired amount of carbohydrate—usually 6 level table-spoons of dextrose. The solution is brought to a boil and allowed to cool, after which the contents of one can of formula base is added. Terminal sterilization is not recommended for this product. Cho-free formula is supplied as a pack of ten 13-ounce cans of liquid concentrate and two 1 ounce cans of dextrose.

13. Sustagen. This formula provides a complete diet or extra nutritional support for the ill, injured, surgical and convalescent patient, and those with impediments to eating or swallowing. Sustagen is made from whole and non-fat milk solids, and contains all known essential nutrients. Chocolate flavored Sustagen contains cocoa. Sustagen is supplied as a powder. The standard solution is prepared by mixing equal parts by volume with water. For example, three cups of Sustagen powder mixed with three cups of water makes about a quart.

14. Skimmed Milk. Powdered skimmed milk (non-fat dry milk) is just as nutritious as liquid skimmed milk. Directions for mixing it are on the container. Skimmed milk is used in the treatment of diarrhea, and recommended for obesity. Fortified skimmed milk with added vitamins is available, but I see no purpose for its existence.

15. Goat's Milk. Goat's milk is worth a try where other formulas have failed to help an allergic child. However, it may be difficult to obtain.

16. No Milk or Milk Substitutes. In some cases milk and milk substitutes are not tolerated at all. The infant can still grow and develop normally. Milk and its substitutes are not the perfect food. Calcium drops may be prescribed.

G

GAGGING AND VOLUNTARY VOMITING

The gagger can usually swallow lumps of food, but resents having it pushed into his throat. To cure gagging let the child feed himself, don't force him. Go slow in changing from strained food. Some children have such sensitive throats that they need to stay on strained foods much longer than the average child.

Most young children can vomit at will. This is likely to happen when they are angry with their parents. If a child expresses his anger openly he may be afraid of the consequences. Therefore, he uses a safe means of expressing his feelings. The child sees that cleaning up the vomitus annoys the parent. He has now evened the score in a safe way. Do not let the child control you through vomiting as long as reasonable standards have been set. They must be enforced in spite of the child's behavior.

GASOLINE—ACCIDENTAL INGESTION

If a child accidentally swallows a petroleum product, such as gasoline or kerosene, *do not pump the stomach out or induce vomiting.* Small amounts of petroleum products or their fumes may cause enough irritation to the lung tissue to lead to pneumonia. If this happens it is called a chemical pneumonia because there is actual destruction of the lung tissue. The diagnosis is confirmed by X ray. I am always astonished that by the time the child is examined an X ray of the chest will demonstrate any changes that are going to take place. There is no correlation between the seriousness of the problem and the amount of petroleum products ingested. If a chemical pneumonia is present, as proven by X rays, hospitalization for observation and treatment is recommended. High fever is apt to develop which is difficult to control. Respiratory distress may occur later. The signs and symptoms of respiratory distress are sucking in, in the neck, between the ribs, under the rib cage and moving in and out of the nose as the child breathes. Antibiotics are given in an effort to prevent secondary infection. Complete recovery usually requires one to two weeks; in severe cases scar tissue may remain in the lung.

If no chemical pneumonia is present as proven by X ray, the child may be safely sent home without medication. He probably did not swallow or inhale the suspected petroleum product. Obviously, the best treatment is prevention. Ideally, all petroleum products should be kept under lock and key. They certainly should not be kept in the garage or any place within a child's reach.

158

GASTRITIS (SEE ALSO VOMITING IN INFANCY—SPITTING)

Gastritis is an infection of the stomach. Vomiting is the major symptom. Fever is seldom present. A viral infection is the usual cause of gastritis, but salmonellosis is not uncommon in older children. (See Food Poisoning.)

Treatment is influenced by the age of the patient. A child's body is composed of a greater per cent of water than an adult's body. Thus, the child (especially a younger child) who vomits for the same length of time is more apt to become dehydrated than an adult. The principles of therapy are complete rest for the gastro-intestinal tract, and the prevention of dehydration. A program applicable to all children regardless of age is given below:

1. Rest the stomach completely for four hours. Give nothing to eat or drink.

2. Following this, start small frequent sips of flat Coke or flat ginger ale at room temperature. Start with an ounce an hour and gradually increase the amount offered as long as there is no more vomiting. If flat Coke or ginger ale is not available, or refused, weak tea may be substituted. Avoid water as children notoriously vomit it for no apparent reason.

3. After clear liquids have been retained for twelve hours, offer one-half strength boiled, skimmed milk. Boil the skimmed milk for twenty minutes and let it cool. Skimmed milk is used because of its low fat content.

4. After twenty-four hours offer simple solids such as cereal, Jello-O, broth, dry toast, or cottage cheese.

5. Late in the second day, full strength skimmed milk may be given.

6. On the third day the diet may be gradually increased, but avoid fatty and heavy foods. Employ the principle of small, frequent feedings.

7. By the fourth or fifth day a regular diet may be eaten. A good response on the part of the patient to the above diet restrictions followed by additional vomiting usually means that the diet restrictions should be continued for a longer period of time.

If vomiting persists beyond twenty-four hours in spite of the above measures, the child should be seen by his physician. Specific

159

medication for vomiting in the form of an injection or suppositories is available. If dehydration is suspected at any time, consult your physician immediately. Dehydration is discussed under the heading Acidosis.

The "bug" causing gastritis frequently invades the intestines, causing diarrhea which compounds the problem. To learn how much additional responsibility to assume, see Diarrhea.

GERMAN MEASLES (RUBELLA)

Because of the frequent occurrence of cataracts, congenital heart disease, hearing loss, mental retardation and other malformations in offspring of mothers infected with German measles in the first six months of pregnancy, all pregnant women must make every effort to avoid this disease. If there is a known exposure or even a questionable exposure, gamma globulin should be given in an effort to prevent German measles. If a pregnant woman, in spite of these precautions, develops German measles during the first six months of pregnancy, therapeutic abortion should be considered. Among women who have rubella in the first three months of pregnancy, approximately seventeen per cent of their offspring have congenital defects. This figure is lowered to approximately ten per cent of the offspring among women who have rubella during the second three months of pregnancy. Of course, if the expectant mother had German measles as a child there is no need for concern; lifetime immunity is the rule.

A. Signs and Symptoms.　German measles begins with a flat, red rash that lasts for approximately three days. There is a simultaneous onset of fever. The glands in the back of the neck become markedly swollen. Feel them yourself. This distinctive sign helps differentiate German measles from other types of febrile illnesses with a rash.

B. Etiology (Cause).　A virus.

C. Treatment.　No specific treatment is available since antibiotics are of no value in a viral infection.

D. Incubation Period.　Ten to twenty-one days—usually eighteen.

E. Period of Communicability.　The disease is communicable just before and during the first few days of recognized illness.

160

F. School Attendance. Isolation of school contacts is not required. The patient may return to school when he has been without fever for forty-eight hours.

G. Prevention. See Immunizations.

H. Complications. German measles is a mild illness in childhood, without complications.

GROWING PAINS

Growing pains are dull quasi-rheumatic pains of varying degree occurring in the limbs, mostly at night, or when the patient is not occupied with play. Children's muscles and bones are growing so rapidly that there is bound to be a pull or tug here and there, causing cramps, particularly in the calves of the legs. Muscle strains, continuous exercise, poor posture, flat feet and weak ankles may also cause growing pains, but don't confuse them with the pain of arthritis or rheumatic fever. These latter diseases are extremely rare.

Aspirin is usually sufficient to control the pain and this in itself proves that there is nothing seriously wrong. Growing pains that occur on a regular basis may require treatment with aspirin regularly for a number of weeks. If the pain persists, a complete physical examination, possibly including X rays and laboratory studies, is indicated.

GROWTH AND DEVELOPMENT—EVALUATION OF

Each baby is an individual unto himself. His growth and development should not be compared with his brother's and sister's, nor to the neighbor's children. Illustrated here is a diagram of the normal distribution curve along which growth and development takes place.

The 25th percentile for weight means that 75 per cent of the children of the same age will weigh more than he does and 25 per cent will weigh less. The 75th percentile for weight means that 25 per cent of the children of the same age will weigh more than he does and 75 per cent will weigh less. The presence of your baby in the 10th percentile or 90th percentile does not indicate that anything is wrong. If a baby's growth and development falls at either end of this distribution curve, it is not average, but still within normal limits.

The percentile into which your baby falls at birth will probably remain constant in spite of growth and development. This is frequently charted and if a marked change occurs diagnostic studies may be indicated. One of the most important reasons for monthly

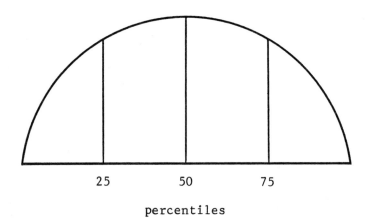

25   50   75

percentiles

well-baby visits is to allow your physician to evaluate your baby's growth and development. This is best done on a continuing basis, and the evaluation must take into consideration all his abilities. For example, a two and one-half year old that does not walk and talk may be perfectly normal. The average age at which to look for specific development is given below. If parents still have doubts they should consult their doctor.

The American Academy of Pediatrics has recommended to physicians the Denver Developmental Screening Test. It is a test that is intended to detect developmental delays. It is administered to the so-called normal child at one year of age as a screening procedure. It is not an intelligence test. The test helps detect hearing loss, minor brain damage and other conditions that are not obvious to either the doctor or parent.

A. The Newborn. The baby sucks, swallows and roots at birth. Rooting means that when the infant smells milk he turns his head to find the source, and that when the cheek is touched by a smooth object, his mouth turns towards the object and his lips open as if to grasp a nipple. Purposeless movements are characteristic of this age. A sneezing reflex is present. A newborn baby can immediately tell light from dark, but he cannot focus clearly enough to recognize people. He distinguishes people by the way they handle him and talk to him.

B. First Month. In general, an infant's motor development takes place from head to toe.

1. He will be able to hold his head up while lying on his stomach.
2. He responds to loud noises.
3. He will flinch at a bright light.
4. He learns to recognize familiar voices.
5. He can taste and smell.
6. He begins to make small throaty sounds.
7. The tonic neck reflex is present. It is characterized by three components:
   (a) the head is turned far to the side;
   (b) one arm is extended on the same side;
   (c) the other arm is bent close to the shoulder.
8. His hands will clench a rattle on contact, but he immediately drops it.
9. When placed in a supported sitting position his head sags forward and the back is evenly rounded.
10. When pulled to the sitting position there is marked lagging of the head.
11. He can move around a little bit, enough to squirm to the corner of the crib.

C. Second Month.

1. He will look at objects.
2. He follows a moving person.
3. He may smile.
4. He makes cooing sounds.
5. He makes single vowel sounds, such as "ah," "eh," "uh."
6. He may be able to grasp a rattle for a short period of time.
7. When he is held he will have control of his neck; it will jerk and bob around, but it will no longer sag forward.

D. Third Month.

1. Head control is markedly improved.
2. He will focus on brightly colored objects and will follow their movements from side to side.

163

3. Salivation becomes active. This is confused with teething by many parents.
4. He will definitely respond to you. Example—when you smile, he will probably coo and smile back.
5. He will raise his chest by pushing up on his arms.
6. In sitting, however, his back is still rounded.
7. Thrashing movements of the arms and legs are common.
8. He may choose a favorite position for sleeping.

E. **Fourth Month.**   The baby's individual personality now becomes apparent. Talk to your baby as he learns to talk by imitation.
1. He will turn his head toward voices.
2. He becomes skilled at focusing his eyes on brightly colored objects.
3. A laugh has developed.
4. There is the beginning of coordination between his eyes and body movements.
5. He looks down at the table top and at his hands.
6. The fingers touch and play with each other.
7. He may discover he can use fingers separately.
8. He regards a rattle in his hand.
9. His hands engage in front of him.
10. There is exploration of his surroundings.
11. When held upright, he will extend his legs and support some weight.
12. He will sit propped up for ten to fifteen minutes. This will not hurt his back. This fear probably originated when rickets was common.
13. He anticipates feeding on sight of food.
14. He is on the verge of rolling over.

F. **Fifth Month.**   He discovers new things about his environment and his own body.
1. Everything automatically goes into the mouth.
2. There is much drooling.
3. He talks to himself when alone.
4. He drops a toy and will follow it with his eyes.
5. He may try to catch moving objects between his hands.
6. He pulls at his clothes.
7. He can sit erect with support. His back is now straighter.

8. He will roll over for the first time. CAUTION: The baby will probably roll over for the first time when you least expect it. Never leave the baby unguarded on a bed, or on any surface from which he can fall.
9. He may appear afraid of strangers because he recognizes the difference between familiar and unfamiliar people.

G. Sixth Month.

1. He will lift his chest up completely, and support himself on his hands and knees.
2. He will grasp objects and possibly transfer an object from one hand to the other.
3. He will possibly pick up objects from the crib.
4. He will move toward objects.
5. He may object when he loses a toy or is left alone. This represents an increased interest in the world around him.
6. He is more sociable, he will look up from what he is doing when people enter the room.

H. Sixth to Ninth Month.

1. He lifts his head while lying on his back.
2. He puts his toes into his mouth.
3. He will say certain words such as "ma-ma" and "da-da."
4. He reaches with one hand.
5. He will transfer a ring from one hand to the other.
6. He will bang a bell.
7. He will pull himself up alone.
8. He will be able to sit alone.
9. He will be able to go from a sitting to a lying down position.
10. The ability to creep usually develops after six months of age. The baby who creeps well may be a late walker if he is satisfied with his ability to move around. Some babies never creep, but only sit until they can stand, and then walk.
11. He will talk to his toys, chew toys and will persistently reach for toys out of reach.
12. Placed before a mirror, he will smile and pat the glass.

I. Ninth to Twelfth Month.

1. He will stand with or without support.
2. He develops the ability to pick up things between the thumb and forefinger. This is called prehensile ability. It is the most useful way of using the hand.

165

3. He will probably start walking. Some babies, however, will not walk until they are two or three years of age and this is not necessarily abnormal.
4. He will show more independence.
5. He may insist upon holding his spoon at meals.
6. He will drink from a cup.
7. He may be reluctant to go to sleep because he does not want to be separated from his parents.
8. He will begin to learn the meaning of the word "No" and to understand simple commands.
9. He imitates sounds, i.e., cough.
10. He responds to his name.
11. He will roll or throw a ball.
12. He will offer a ball to you, but not release it.
13. He will grasp a bell by its handle.
14. He will pull on a string.
15. He will relinquish a toy on request.
16. He will attempt to build a tower with blocks without success.
17. He will cooperate in dressing.
18. He will play "patacake" and "bye-bye."
19. He will place two cubes together.
20. He will place a cube in a cup.
21. He will try to insert a pellet in a bottle, with success.

J. Twelve to Eighteen Months.
1. He will use a spoon well.
2. He will use groups of words with gestures.
3. He will sit in a small chair without assistance.
4. He seldom falls when walking.
5. He will climb stairs.
6. He will run.
7. He hurls a ball.
8. He will turn pages of a book.
9. He will put blocks in a hole.
10. He will imitate strokes with a crayon.
11. He identifies one picture.
12. He builds a tower of three blocks.
13. He pulls a toy.
14. On command he will put a toy on a chair.

166

15. He plays with and carries about a stuffed animal.
16. He hands the empty dish to his mother.
17. He fills a cup with cubes.
18. He dumps pellets from a bottle.

K. Two Years.

1. He points to his eyes, nose and mouth.
2. He imitates circular strokes.
3. He kicks a ball.
4. He turns pages singly.
5. He identifies three to five pictures.
6. He feeds his stuffed animal.
7. He builds a tower of seven blocks.
8. He aligns cubes.
9. He uses three to four word sentences.
10. He asks for food and drink.
11. He asks to go to the toilet.
12. He verbalizes his immediate experience, referring to himself by name.
13. He carries out simple commands on request.
14. He often squats to play on the floor.
15. His play includes domestic mimicry.
16. He engages in parallel play with other children, doing the same things nearby, but not with mutual cooperation.

L. Three Years.

1. He copies a circle.
2. He matches three color forms.
3. He builds a tower of ten blocks.
4. He kicks a ball well.
5. He jumps on both feet and can jump down from a height of five feet.
6. He can walk on his tip toes.
7. He pulls on his shoe.
8. He stands on one foot momentarily.
9. He peddles a bicycle.
10. He unbuttons his clothing.
11. He pours liquid from a pitcher to a glass.
12. He feeds himself with little spilling.
13. His vocabulary contains many words.
14. He gives his last name.

15. He gives his sex.
16. He speaks in well formed simple sentences, using plurals.
17. He repeats three digits.
18. He may not wet his bed.

H

HEADACHE

Headache goes along with almost any childhood illness. Headache affecting the forehead or located behind the eyes is particularly common with viral infections. If headache is relieved by aspirin, parents can assume that it is not too serious. Recurrent headaches that get progressively worse, that are not relieved by aspirin, and are located in the back or possibly on the side of the head, deserve consultation with a physician.

HEAD INJURY—CONCUSSION AND CONTUSIONS AND SKULL FRACTURES

Children frequently fall out of bed or stumble and hit their heads. If the blow is hard enough a lump will appear. The lump (hematoma) is caused by bleeding from a broken blood vessel under the skin. The swelling stops enlarging when the pressure in the closed space under the skin increases enough to constrict the blood vessel. *The swelling itself is of no major concern.* The important question is whether there is injury to the underlying brain. To answer this question the dynamics involved in a blow to the head must be understood. The brain is surrounded by the bony skull for protection. Think of a shoe in a shoe box. If the shoe box is dropped, the shoe may vibrate, hitting one side of the box, bounce off, hit the other side of the box and vibrate back and forth a number of times before coming to rest. This same principle applies to the brain. When the skull is hit with enough force the brain underneath may vibrate back and forth causing an injury. An X ray of the skull is obtained in all cases of head injury to rule out a fracture.

168

If a child has a lump on his head without evidence of any injury to the underlying brain and the X ray of the skull is normal, he may be safely cared for at home. However, he must be watched for delayed and persistent vomiting. Parents always seem to want to keep such a child awake. *There is no reason not to let him sleep. He needs only to be awakened occasionally to make sure that he is not in a coma.*

If X rays demonstrate a fractured skull, do not panic. A skull when fractured, i.e., the bone has a crack in it, will heal perfectly well. Physicians are not concerned about a skull fracture by itself. *The important considerations are whether there is underlying damage to the brain or if any part of the bony skull is pushed down into the brain.* If part of the skull is depressed, surgical intervention is necessary to elevate it. Fortunately, most skull fractures are uncomplicated. Even so, the child must be hospitalized and observed for complications.

A concussion is characterized by transitory unconsciousness without evidence of structural brain damage. The signs and symptoms of a concussion, all of which need not be present, include:

1. Headache.
2. Drowsiness.
3. Slight disorientation.
4. Pallor.
5. Vomiting.
6. Amnesia (loss of memory concerning the event).
7. Loss of consciousness of some degree. This may be a fleeting feeling of being dazed or the patient may not respond to the spoken voice for several minutes to several hours.
8. Dizziness.
9. The neurological examination is within normal limits. The general picture is that of a person in shock. I want to emphasize that a concussion is not seen on an X ray. It is a clinical diagnosis made in retrospect after it is clear that the patient has no indication of damage to the brain. It is impossible to assert in the acute stages of head injury while the patient is still unconscious.

Any child with a concussion should be hospitalized. The treatment consists of strict bed rest with frequent determination of the patient's pulse, blood pressure, respiration and pupil size. Does the patient remain oriented as to time, place and person? Does the patient continue to move all extremities? If any significant change occurs in these signs, or in the patient's general condition, the physician will be on the lookout for complications.

The child with a concussion should remain in the hospital for at least forty-eight to seventy-two hours. Hemorrhage into the brain may occur as a delayed reaction. With significant hemorrhage one pupil becomes larger than the other. The above may sound quite frightening to you as a parent, but let me assure you that this complication is extremely rare. The vast majority of cases recover within a few days to several weeks.

A contusion is characterized by hemorrhage into the brain substance. The symptoms are similar to those of concussion but the unconsciousness is usually prolonged, and convulsions may occur. Neurological examination may reveal evidence of brain damage such as muscle weakness. The spinal fluid (see Spinal Tap) often contains blood.

Parents must learn to be patient when a child sustains a head injury. The nervous system has marvelous recuperative powers, but time is required. A physician cannot really assess if there has been permanent damage following a head injury for at least six months.

HEARING (DEAFNESS)

Hearing is the faculty or sense by which sound is perceived. The ability to hear enough to develop speech needs to be determined as soon as possible after birth, so that those children with impaired hearing may receive the maximum amount of help possible. The ability to hear may be routinely tested for in the hospital nursery, or at the first well-baby visit in your physician's office. This is done by projecting a certain sound. The baby is supposed to respond with a startle (moro) reflex. A startle reflex is defined as raising of the hands and feet. This may be accompanied by slight shaking. This does not mean that the baby has perfect hearing, but it does tell us that he is able to hear those sounds of a certain frequency and intensity that are most important for the development of speech.

A child who can respond to directions has his hearing tested by means of an audiogram. An audiometer projects certain frequencies of sound at different intensities. The child then indicates if he hears these sounds. This can be done by instructing the child to drop a peg in a can when he hears the tone. Since this is a highly specialized and expensive piece of equipment that should be used in a sound-proof room for accuracy, a referral to an audiologist and speech pathologist is usually necessary. Testing hearing by the use of whispered numbers or the tick of a clock is unscientific and inadequate.

An audiologist is a person holding a master's or doctorate in the science of hearing. He administers and interprets hearing tests. He advises a patient regarding the selection of a hearing aid and other rehabilitative services for the deaf and hard of hearing, including educational placement.

A speech pathologist is a person holding a master's or doctorate in the profession dedicated to the rehabilitation of speech and language problems. He evaluates speech and language skills and, when appropriate, plans and executes a program of rehabilitation.

Much can be done to help the newborn with inadequate hearing to develop speech. The sooner a hearing aid is worn, the better. Hearing aids are small and light. If worn in the ear, the part containing the battery, transistor and microphone may be hidden behind the ear and covered by hair. Generally speaking, the type of hearing aid worn behind the ear is more satisfactory than an aid worn around the neck. There is better spacial orientation because when the child turns his head the microphone also turns.

The educational process must be started as soon as possible in children hard of hearing. These children are not "deaf, dumb and blind." Our own ignorance originally led to this phrase. The problem in educating these children is not lack of ability, but the fact that they require many more repetitions of the same word in order to learn it than the child with normal hearing. It is difficult to teach these children concepts, because they are difficult to put into words. For example, how do you teach the concept of danger? It is much easier for the child to learn when he can use some of his other senses—sight, touch, taste and smell. Children with hearing impairment should start formal instruction as soon as possible. Ideally their education should be continuous throughout the year. Many children with a mild or moderate hearing loss can function well in the usual school situation, providing they obtain additional speech therapy. If at all possible these children should not be relegated to a special school for the deaf. A child who is constantly around other children with severe hearing loss will not talk distinctly. Many children with impaired hearing lip read. There is nothing wrong with this.

If the hearing loss is severe, parents have to accept the fact that sign language will be necessary. The parents of a child with hearing loss are bound to feel guilty. I want to emphasize that nothing they did or did not do caused any nerve deafness. Their feelings should be discussed with a trained clinical psychologist or psychiatrist.

The commonest cause of acquired hearing loss is recurrent ear infections that have not responded to therapy. When your child has otitis media make sure that there is adequate follow-up to prevent this. (See Otitis Media.)

Prolonged exposure to rock'n'roll music may eventually cause hearing impairments. Live rock'n'roll band rehearsal creates 120 to 130 decibels—the Saturn moon rocket from the press box only 120 decibels. Noise levels above 100 decibels may do permanent damage to the ears. Safe maximum standards for electronic amplifiers in teenage clubs and discotheques need to be established.

HEART MURMURS

A heart murmur may be thought of as a continuous sound heard through a stethoscope such as the wind blowing in a tree or of low indistinct voices. The murmur may be produced by the abnormal opening and closing of the valves, the abnormal flow of blood in the chambers of the heart and the great vessels, or by the passage of blood through deformed valves. A systolic murmur occurs when the heart contracts. A diastolic murmur occurs when the heart relaxes. There are three causes of heart murmurs:

1. Functional or so-called meaningless, physiologic normal, harmless murmurs.
2. Congenital heart disease.
3. Acquired heart disease such as rheumatic fever.

Parents should not become frightened when they are told their child has a heart murmur, because *by far the functional or physiologic heart murmur is the most common.* It has been said that if a child's heart is checked carefully and frequently enough, a heart

172

murmur will be heard sometime in his life. A child that has a functional heart murmur has no signs and symptoms of heart disease. There is no blueness, shortness of breath, squatting, repeated attacks of pneumonia or retarded growth and development. The murmur itself may be so characteristically functional in its location and quality to the physician that a complete cardiac workup including electrocardiogram and chest X ray is not always necessary when the physician's clinical findings are correlated with a normal history. A child need not lead a sheltered life or have any restrictions placed upon him when an innocent murmur is present. The parents should listen carefully to what the doctor says. In spite of assurance that a functional murmur is not cause for alarm, some parents insist on overprotecting their child. The child in turn becomes indoctrinated with the idea that he has heart trouble and leads a restrained life. Many children with heart trouble have to take precautions, but it is just as bad when a child who really does not have heart disease is forced to live with the idea that he has. Murmurs from congenital heart disease are present at birth or shortly thereafter. (See Congenital Heart Disease.) Murmurs that develop from rheumatic fever are accompanied by other signs and symptoms. (See Rheumatic Fever.)

HEAT RASH—PRICKLY HEAT (MILIARIA RUBRA)

Heat rash is a common condition that affects almost all babies at some time or other. It may even occur in the winter. Prickly heat is usually located around the neck and over the shoulders and chest, but the entire body may be involved, causing the parents unnecessary concern. The rash is red, and flat to slightly raised.

This harmless but irritating rash arises from obstruction of the sweat pores and is seen with extensive sweating. Treatment consists of the following measures:

1. Avoid overdressing the baby. Dress your baby as you would dress yourself. If you are too hot, assume the baby is too hot.
2. Bathe the baby frequently in cool water or apply alcohol to the skin three or four times a day. Follow this by the application of a powder that helps absorb perspiration. My favorite is Ammens Powder, which is available in the drugstore without a prescription. Many other powders are satisfactory. Ask your doctor or pharma

cist which one he recommends. Cornstarch may work well. Frequently, the same medication does not always work.

3. Keep the house cool by using fans or air conditioning. CAUTION: Do not let the air blow directly on the baby since this may cause chilling.

4. Avoid oily skin preparations.

5. Avoid sun exposure.

If the baby fails to respond to the above measures, consult your physician. In severe or resistant cases, cortisone ointment is marvelous.

Unfortunately, the struggle against heat rash is often constant, particularly if your baby has sensitive skin.

HEMANGIOMAS (BIRTHMARKS)

Hemangiomas are collections of superficial blood vessels that vary in size and shape from fractions of an inch to very large areas. They are not cancerous. Very small strawberry or raised red marks are very common in the newborn, particularly on the eyelids and the back of the head.

Hemangiomas will spontaneously disappear, particularly during the first few years of life. As resolution occurs, the center of the hemangioma becomes white. Many physicians have seen hemangiomas covering half the face or the entire diaper area. Even these large hemangiomas disappear spontaneously with patience. Human hands cannot improve upon the cosmetic result nature obtains. The dermatologist need not freeze them, the radiologist need not X-ray them, and the surgeon need not remove them. Since children are naturally cruel to each other, an older child may be teased and picked on. If this occurs, discuss his feelings with him and give him extra support.

HEMOPHILIA

Hemophilia has been classically known as "the disease of kings" because a number of European monarchs were sufferers in centuries past. It is a hereditary bleeding disorder caused by the lack of antihemophiliac globulin which is necessary for blood to clot

174

normally. Various forms of this disease have been discovered; consequently physicians can no longer make the categorical statement that hemophilia occurs only in males. The diagnosis is established by performing special studies on the patient's blood. They are intricate and delicate to do and thus are rarely performed in your physician's office.

The major symptom is bleeding. The slightest cut or bruise is liable to lead to uncontrolled hemorrhage. Since children are always falling, bleeding commonly occurs in their joints, particularly the elbow and knee. Deformities develop if this happens frequently. Of course there is always the possibility of brain hemorrhage, but from a practical standpoint this is extremely rare. Proper treatment must be obtained once hemorrhage starts. In some cases only a pressure bandage is necessary. The parents and child become adept at observing continued bleeding which requires additional treatment, such as fresh-frozen plasma, fresh blood, or concentrated antihemophilic factor. Repeated transfusions with one or more of these agents may be necessary over a period of a few days to prevent additional bleeding. Blood stored in a blood bank is of no value since the antihemophilic factor which stops the bleeding is rapidly destroyed by the passage of time. There are case reports in the literature of hemophiliacs playing football by using frequent injections of the concentrated antihemophilic factor. It is foolish to prove one's masculinity in this way.

The prevention of bleeding is the most important single aspect in the control of this illness. Obviously, hemophilic children need to be protected by wearing splints, by not participating in athletics, and by being extremely careful to avoid falling or other bodily injury. These children will learn how to limit their own activities with guidance from their parents. They should use an electric shaver for shaving. As with any incurable disease, certain attitudes and feelings are going to develop in the child, particularly when he is prohibited from doing many normal things that other children do. However, do not permit him to use his illness for personal gain and gratification. If parents see this occurring, the parents and child should receive adequate help from a physician who is particularly interested in feelings, or from a clinical psychologist or psychiatrist.

Development of an emergency self-treatment technique for hemophilia victims has been forecast. This would utilize a fountain pen sized syringe containing a potent blood clotting substance—a high potency "antihemophilia factor" (AHF).

Since hemophilia is a disease for which there is no cure, proper medical supervision is most important. A good doctor-patient relationship must be maintained. With good care, hemophilic children can certainly grow up, get married and raise a family. With a little bit of luck, good care and sensible treatment, the patient can be expected to live much of his normal life span. Through research a protein in the blood of hemophiliacs that prompts a spleen other then their own to produce antihemophilic factor (AHF) has been discovered. This discovery raises the eventual possibility of spleenic transplants to combat hemophilia.

HEPATITIS—INFECTIOUS

Hepatitis is an infection involving the liver.
A. Signs and Symptoms.

1. Fatigue.
2. Weight loss.
3. Change in the color of the stools and urine.
4. Finally, yellowness (jaundice).

A battery of simple laboratory tests performed on the blood confirms the diagnosis. Many mild cases are never diagnosed because there is no visible jaundice to make the doctor suspicious of the disease.

B. Etiology (Cause).   A virus.

C. Treatment.   Antibiotic is of no value since the infection is viral in origin. Rest is the cornerstone of treatment. Activity may have to be limited for a number of months. The sedimentation rate is a nonspecific blood test of disease activity that enables the physician to accurately follow the course of hepatitis. As long as it remains elevated additional rest is needed. A balanced diet is important.

D. Incubation Period.   Ten to forty days.

E. Period of Communicability.   Not known. It is assumed to be approximately one week, starting a few days before the onset of illness.

F. School Attendance. Not permitted without the approval of your physician.

G. Prevention. Infectious hepatitis may be prevented by the use of gamma globulin. A shot of gamma globulin provides protection for about three weeks. Additional exposure after this time requires another shot.

H. Complications. Permanent liver damage rarely occurs, but it may be progressive in nature.

HERNIA (RUPTURE)

A hernia is considered to be a congenital defect in supporting tissue of the body, allowing the intestine to escape from the abdominal cavity (belly) causing a lump or swelling. A rupture is not caused by excessive crying. If the hernia appears in the scrotum, or by the groin, it is called an inguinal hernia. If the hernia appears about the belly button, it is called an umbilical hernia. Hernias are more commonly found in males and there are some indications that in some families male members show a tendency to develop them.

A. Inguinal Hernia. There are no specific symptoms of uncomplicated hernia. Pain is not present. A lump is usually seen or felt by the mother when she bathes her child. The doctor confirms her diagnosis. Often the lump reduces itself and then reappears. Bilateral hernias are not uncommon. Spontaneous cures are almost unheard of. The wearing of trusses or supports to keep the swelling down is not recommended for children. The treatment of choice is elective surgery. Repair is indicated as soon as possible, with the parent and the physician choosing the time of surgery. This prevents surgical emergencies and complications, such as strangulation. Strangulation occurs if a portion of the bowel becomes caught in the sac of the hernia, resulting in obstruction to the blood supply and possibly death of the bowel. The signs and symptoms of a strangulated inguinal hernia are:

1. Swelling which the doctor cannot reduce (push down).
2. Pain.
3. Vomiting.

177

Immediate surgery must be performed if strangulation occurs. Elective repair also avoids the possibility of vomiting when an anesthetic must be given to a child that has recently eaten. Aspiration of the vomitus into the lungs may cause pneumonia.

Although I have respect for all operations, the repair of a hernia is a relatively simple procedure. The results are excellent. Prolonged hospitalization is not necessary. A child under a year of age will probably be hospitalized only over night. The recurrence of the hernia following surgical repair is extremely unusual, but should not be considered a reflection on the operating surgeon.

B. Umbilical Hernia. Umbilical hernias are present at birth. They may vary in size from that of a dime to a half dollar. An umbilical hernia will increase in size and bulge out when the child is crying or coughing. It is painless and in no way harmful to the child. Umbilical hernias are very common in the Negro race. Conservative treatment is indicated. Taping the hernia early in life is helpful. The swelling should be reduced (pushed down) and the skin drawn together and taped with adhesive. Apply tincture of benzoin to the skin before taping to prevent irritation. It is available in the drugstore without a prescription. Keep the hernia taped until it is considerably smaller—probably a number of months. An umbilical hernia will close spontaneously unless extremely large. It becomes less and less noticeable as the size of the abdominal cavity (belly) increases and as the muscles of the abdominal wall become stronger. Remember that all children are pot-bellied to begin with, thus accentuating the problem. Surgery is rarely necessary. Strangulation of an umbilical hernia is unheard of. Therefore, if surgery is performed in an older child it is for cosmetic reasons.

HICCUPS

Hiccups are caused by air which is swallowed when the baby is fed. Spasms of the diaphragm muscle which separates the chest contents from the abdominal (belly) contents occur. Hiccups are aggravating both to the baby and parent, although they are not painful. Hiccups can usually be relieved by burping the baby. Sometimes a drink of warm water will help.

HIP—CONGENITAL DISLOCATION

Congenital dislocation of the hip means that the long bone of the upper part of the leg called the femur is not properly attached to the pelvis. This is a ball and socket joint; in other words there is a large rounded area on the end of the femur which inserts itself into a socket in the pelvis. In congenital dislocation of the hip, the socket into which the ball fits is not properly developed.

Each time your baby has his well-baby checkup, your physician will take his lower legs and frog them out. The legs are pushed back to the belly and out to the side, creating a 90-degree angle. This examination rules out the presence of a congenitally dislocated hip. If the hip is dislocated, your physician will not be able to frog out your baby's legs. He may also hear a click or feel a snap. Another sign is the lack of symmetrical skin folds in the back of the thighs. One or both hips may be involved. The diagnosis is confirmed by X ray.

The exact cause of congenital dislocation of the hip is unknown, but a heredity factor has been repeatedly observed. It is found approximately seven times more frequently in the female than in the male. It occurs more frequently in certain parts of the world such as southern France and northern Italy. The incidence of congenital dislocation of the hip is one to three cases per thousand births in the United States.

It is imperative that the diagnosis be established to prevent the condition from becoming progressively worse. In early infancy, the only treatment necessary may be keeping the thighs in a frog-like position by using a thickened diaper or pillow. In later infancy, a cast to immobilize the hip may be necessary for a period of six to nine months. Careful observation of the skin around the edges of any cast is necessary to note any irritation. Explore under the cast for any loose objects or food particles which the child may have stuffed there. Every effort must be made to keep the child as active as possible in spite of a cast. Parents cannot let a child regress emotionally and mentally while taking care of a physical defect. Once the condition is corrected there is no recurrence. Most children have an excellent response to therapy. However, if treatment was not begun before the age of three, surgical correction is generally necessary.

179

HIVES

Hives are giant welts that are most uncomfortable due to itching. They are allergic in origin, but frequently the exact cause is unknown. In most cases of hives, without swelling of the lips or hoarseness, give an antihistamine, such as triaminic which is available in the drugstore without a prescription. See Colds for the suggested dosage. For itching apply calamine (Caladryl) lotion. It is available in the drugstore without a prescription.

In severe cases, with swelling of the lips or hoarseness, your physician must be consulted immediately. Hoarseness means that there is some swelling in the airway that could become worse, leading to respiratory distress unless more rapidly acting and more potent medication is used—such as adrenalin and/or cortisone. (See Croup and Asthma and the Allergic Patient.)

HOOK WORMS

Hookworm is a parasitic disease that is not uncommon in the southern part of the United States. Hookworm enters the skin when children go bare footed in soil that is contaminated.

The signs and symptoms are disturbed digestion and blood in the stools. Children with hookworm sometimes develop severe anemia. The diagnosis is confirmed by finding the characteristic eggs in the stool.

Specific treatment is available from your doctor. The drug of choice is tetrachlorethylene. This drug is a safe effective liquid that is administered orally. A light evening meal, preferably liquid, is eaten the night preceding treatment. No breakfast is allowed the following morning. The full amount of the drug is then administered. A single treatment will remove approximately ninety per cent of the hookworms. If eggs are present in the stools two weeks after treatment, a second course may be given.

HOT SOAKS (WET DRESSINGS)

Hot soaks are extremely valuable in the treatment of localized infections such as boils and abscesses. They help the body absorb the pus or localize it into a head. A washcloth is placed in hot water, wrung out and applied over the infected area. It is not necessary to use salt water or epsom salts. When the washcloth is cool, the procedure is repeated. The hotter the child can stand it, the better. Soak the involved area for at least twenty minutes four times a day. The more often this can be done, the more rapid the healing.

HYALINE MEMBRANE DISEASE

Hyaline membrane disease occurs only in the newborn. It affects the lungs and causes difficulty in breathing. At birth the baby has perfectly normal respirations. A few hours later he develops respiratory distress. In mild cases there is a slight increase in the respiratory rate. In severe cases the breathing difficulty is manifested by sucking in under the ribs, between the ribs, in the neck, and in and out flaring movements of the nose. Newborns affected with hyaline membrane disease may breathe as rapidly as one hundred times a minute, and live. Rapid breathing is not necessarily a bad sign as it is an effort by the infant to exchange more air.

Hyaline membrane disease is caused by a membrane that obstructs the exchange of air. The exact conditions that lead to the formation of this membrane are not known. However, it is more frequent in babies born by Caesarian section, babies of diabetic mothers, and prematures. In some cases a chest X ray reveals a typical appearance that is diagnostic.

There is no drug that specifically combats this disease. However, many babies have responded adequately to supportive therapy, including oxygen, fluids and antibiotics. Some infants who survive severe hyaline membrane disease have been shown to have residual scarring of the lungs.

HYDROCELE (SWELLING ABOUT THE TESTICLE)

A hydrocele is a tense collection of fluid about the testicle which may vary in size from day to day. It is not painful. One or both sides may be involved, with one side being bigger than the other. A hydrocele is usually discovered at birth, or shortly thereafter. It may be confused with a hernia (rupture), but can be easily differentiated by holding a flashlight next to the swelling. If the light transluminates, i.e., light is seen through the swelling, a hydrocele is present.

181

Most hydroceles will spontaneously cure themselves by a year of age. Surgery is rarely necessary, unless the hydrocele gets progressively larger or fails to disappear by a year of age. Occasionally, there is an associated hernia which cannot be felt because of the fluid. Of course, all inguinal hernias must be surgically repaired. (See Hernia.)

HYDROCEPHALUS

Hydrocephalus is an accumulation of fluid within the brain that causes rapid enlargement of the head. The head may be normal in size at birth, but enlarges at a rapid rate thereafter. At each well-baby visit during the first year of life your physician will measure the circumference of the baby's head and chest to determine any abnormal enlargement of the head in comparison to the chest. At birth the head circumference is normally larger than the chest, at approximately six months of age they are equal, and thereafter the chest circumference is larger. As the head abnormally enlarges in hydrocephalus, the forehead becomes prominent and the upper eyelids are drawn upward. In severe cases, it becomes impossible to close the eyelids completely. As the infant grows he will not develop head control because of its large size and increased weight. In progressive unarrested cases, both physical and mental development lag. The child becomes sleepy and dull. The cry is often high pitched and the infant is restless and irritable. The arms and legs may become rigid and convulsions occasionally occur. Vomiting is frequent.

Hydrocephalus is caused by an excessive accumulation of cerebral spinal fluid because there is obstruction to its flow. In certain amounts this fluid is normal as its function is to bathe our nervous system. Hydrocephalus is usually the result of a congenital abnormality, but may result from a tumor or infection. X rays confirm the diagnosis made on the basis of a proper history and physical examination. Special X-ray techniques, such as the injection of dye or air into the central nervous system, are performed when indicated.

Treatment consists of surgical excision of any obstruction to the flow of cerebral spinal fluid if it is accessible and amenable to an operation. Unfortunately, the structural abnormalities are not accessible to a direct surgical approach in most cases. Therefore,

182

treatment is directed at reducing the volume of the cerebral spinal fluid present in the brain. Nine different surgical procedures have been developed to cope with this problem. They are called shunting operations. Although shunting procedures provide some temporary success, they frequently meet with failure after functioning for a short period of time. Your physician will decide the best course of action for each child.

Spontaneous arrest of the disease process has been reported but this is extremely rare. Many parents have the unfounded fear that the child's head may burst. This will never occur. At worst, there may be a gradual leak of spinal fluid through the scalp.

A child with hydrocephalus should be treated as normally as possible, be provided with toys and tender loving care. Within a short period of time the parents and physician will be able to tell if the child's hydrocephalus is progressive with resultant mental deterioration. With progressive disease, there is little hope of the child being able to take care of his routine needs at any age. Providing special care in a nursing home equipped for retarded children or in a state institution should be seriously considered. Hydrocephalus is frequently associated with other congenital abnormalities of the central nervous system that are incompatible with life.

HYDRONEPHROSIS

Hydronephrosis means that dilation of the kidneys and/ureters is present. The ureters, which are similar to long tubes, carry urine from the kidneys to the bladder. Hydronephrosis is caused by obstruction to the urinary tract. This may be due to an abnormal blood vessel crossing the ureter, a kink in the ureter, a mass pressing on the ureter, an overdeveloped bladder muscle or abnormal development. If the obstruction is in the bladder, the dilation of the kidneys and ureters occurs on both sides. If the obstruction is above the bladder, the dilation occurs only on one side unless each side is separately obstructed.

The only symptom may be a urinary tract infection. (See Cystitis and Pyelonephritis.) Therefore, if your child has a urinary tract infection, an X ray of the kidneys must be considered. It is a pity to miss this diagnosis by neglecting to take X rays. One can rationalize and say that the chances of your child having hydronephrosis is slight, even if a kidney tract infection is present. This is true, but medicine cannot be practiced on a statistical basis. It is important to make the diagnosis as early as possible in order to prevent and limit damage to the kidneys. Many of these obstructions can be surgically cured.

HYPERTHYROIDISM (OVERACTIVE THYROID)

Hyperthyroidism means there is over activity of the thyroid gland located in the neck. The signs and symptoms are:

1. Rapid pulse.
2. Elevated blood pressure.
3. Tremors.
4. Emotional instability.
5. Hyperactivity.
6. Bulging of the eyes.
7. Accelerated growth.
8. Loss of weight.

Hyperthyroidism is due to over-production of the thyroid hormone. The basal metabolic rate (BMR) used to be widely used to confirm the diagnosis. This was a test that determined the patient's metabolism when he was in a resting state. The obvious difficulty of establishing such a state lead to many inaccuracies. This test has been replaced by more sophisticated blood tests. An interesting diagnostic test is a machine that times our ankle (Achilles) reflex since the speed of our reflexes is affected by the thyroid hormone.

Specific drug therapy is available. The response is remarkably good. Radioactive iodine is used to treat some selective cases. Occasionally, surgical excision is indicated, followed by the use of drugs. The best treatment for your child will be determined by your physician. With proper treatment a normal and healthy life is to be expected.

HYPOGAMMAGLOBULINEMIA

A patient recovering from infection acquires natural immunity by the production of antibodies that protect him from contracting that same illness again for a period of time, and in some cases for-

184

ever. Hypogammaglobulinemia means there is a *deficiency* in gamma globulin—a protein found in our blood. Hence, our body cannot produce or store enough antibodies to protect us properly from bacterial infections. Interestingly enough, the patient's ability to fight viral infections is not affected. This is not cancer of the blood.

The outstanding symptom of this disease is recurrent infections and the inability to fight infections properly. To make the diagnosis your physician must be clinically suspicious of any child who has recurrent infections. Is there an underlying cause? The diagnosis is confirmed by a special blood test called an electrophoretic pattern.

Fortunately, most patients with hypogammaglobulinemia out-grow it with adequate treatment. Frequent infections are prevented by routine injections of gamma globulin every three to four weeks. The clinical response of the patient correlated with the measurement of his gamma globulin level permits appropriate adjustment of dosage. The approximate duration of therapy is six months to one year. Parents are happy to see their child stay well once treatment is started. Many parents have reported to me that their child becomes irritable two or three days before the next dose of gamma globulin is due. This may be the individual child saying that he needs more gamma globulin at the moment. Giving it a few days early will not hurt, but be sure never to be late. If a bacterial infection occurs, specific antibiotic treatment is indicated. Therefore, it is best to consult your physician at the first sign of illness. Avoid waiting two or three days as you might in a child that can normally fight infection.

HYPOSPADIAS

The external meatus through which males void is normally located in the middle of the head of the penis. Hypospadias means that the external meatus is located abnormally on the underside of the head of the penis or even in the shaft of the penis. This is a congenital abnormality that presents itself at birth. It is advisable to consider an X ray of the entire urinary system to rule out any other defects in development. Children born with hypospadias should not be circumcised in order that the skin may be saved and used for surgical repair of the penis later in life. Surgical treatment

185

is usually instituted at about two years of age. Occasionally more than one operation is necessary. Until surgical correction, the end of the penis may appear crooked.

HYPOTHYROIDISM (UNDERACTIVE THYROID)

Hypothyroidism means there is under activity of the thyroid gland located in the neck. It is the commonest endocrine disorder in children. In congenital cases, it is important to make the diagnosis as soon as possible after birth so that mental deficiency may be prevented with proper therapy. The earliest signs in the infant are:

1. A good baby—
   a. never cries;
   b. sleeps through the night;
   c. falls asleep on the bottle.
2. Sucks poorly.
3. Always feels cold.
4. Constipation in spite of treatment.

Parents may be more familiar with the name "cretin" which is a term used in congenital cases that did not receive therapy early enough. A cretin is characterized by physical deformity, dwarfism and idiocy. In the acquired type of hypothyroidism that occurs after birth, mental deficiency is not a threat.

The signs and symptoms of the acquired type are:

1. Swelling of the skin tissues.
2. Enlarged tongue.
3. Cool dry skin.
4. Coarse hair.
5. Delayed development of the teeth.
6. Poor muscle tone with associated constipation.
7. Easy fatigability.
8. Slow pulse.
9. Decrease in blood pressure.
10. Subnormal body temperature with intolerance to cold.
11. Obesity.

Hypothyroidism is due to a deficiency in the thyroid hormone produced by the thyroid gland. The basal metabolic rate (BMR) was at one time widely used to confirm the diagnosis. This was a test that determined the patient's metabolism when he was in a resting state. The obvious difficulty of establishing such a state lead to many inaccuracies. This test has been replaced by more sophisticated blood tests. An interesting diagnostic test is a machine that times our ankle (Achilles) reflex since the speed of our reflexes are affected by the thyroid hormone.

Treatment consists of placing the patient on thyroid hormone. The response is remarkably good. A normal life span is to be expected.

I

IMMUNIZATIONS

Many parents are negligent in obtaining routine immunizations for their children. They no longer hear about whooping cough and diphtheria, and therefore feel that immunizations against these diseases are not necessary. However, when enough of the population is not protected against these diseases there will be an epidemic in the unprotected population sooner or later.

Your physician will keep a record of all immunizations given to your child, which is always available to you or to any other physician. However, the parents should maintain a separate record of all immunizations given their baby. Take this with you on vacation. That way, if your child should have an accident, your standby physician will know whether any booster immunizations are necessary. The specific order in which your physician desires to give the routine immunizations at well-baby checkups is up to him. Some physicians will start immunizations at a slightly later date than others. Regardless, the receiving of proper immunization is very important. I do not believe that children under a year of age should be immunized without an appropriate physical examination since the possibility of illness, without obvious symptoms, always exists.

Reactions consisting mainly of fever are common with most immunizations. Tempra or tylenol with aspirin may be given. (See Tempra, Tylenol, Aspirin.) Of course, the suggested immunizations discussed below are subject to modification as further advances are made in medical knowledge.

1. DPT—Diphtheria, Whooping Cough, Tetanus. The "P" stands for pertussis which is the medical term for whooping cough. Protection against these diseases is given simultaneously in the same syringe; thus, they are also known as three-in-one shots. Three injections are given a month apart. If because of illness or some inadvertent reason more than a month or two elapses between any of the DPT shots, the protection afforded will still be adequate, provided enough vaccine is given to put the child back on the standard immunization schedule. The first booster shot is given a year later. Thereafter, a booster DPT injection should be given every three years up to the age of ten.

Children over the age of ten are not routinely immunized against whooping cough. If it should be considered advisable, a single vaccine is used.

For practical purposes protection against diphtheria stimulated by immunization is allowed to wane in children over the age of ten unless the child has been exposed to a specific case. Upon exposure, a Schick test is performed to determine the patient's susceptibility. If the patient is immune, no reaction will occur. If the patient is susceptible, an area of reddish brown discoloration appears at the site of injection. Then proper immunization is given. Before administering diphtheria toxoid, patients over the age of ten are always tested for sensitivity to it.

If a child aged ten or older has never been immunized against tetanus, two or three single injections at monthly intervals are given, depending on whether the material used is alum-precipitated or fluid tetanus toxoid. Tetanus boosters should be kept up throughout a person's entire life—every three to five years, even when there have been no injuries. If a dirty cut or wound is sustained, the patient should receive a tetanus booster unless the most recent immunization has been within the last year. In case of injury and no previous immunization against tetanus, tetanus antitoxin prepared from horse serum is administered. Antitoxin may cause a serious allergic reaction. Therefore, the patient must always be skin tested

188

to rule out allergy to this material before its use. Fortunately, human tetanus antitoxin called homotet is now available in case the patient is allergic to horse serum. Since an antitoxin provides only temporary immunity—in other words, the immunity is passively transferred —routine immunization against tetanus will still be necessary to stimulate adequate active immunity in the individual patient to protect him from the illness on a long-term basis.

Fussiness or fever of 101 to 102 degrees is a common reaction to any of these shots. These symptoms do not usually last for more than forty-eight or seventy-two hours and are easily controlled with aspirin and tempra or tylenol. DPT injections do not precipitate colds or coughs. Such an occurrence is strictly coincidental.

2. German Measles (Rubella). The vaccine against German measles probably provides permanent lifetime immunity, without booster injections. The only side effects are a mild rash around the site of injection and an occasional transient joint pain. The live rubella vaccine is recommended for boys and girls between the age of one year and puberty. A history of rubella illness is usually not reliable enough to exclude children from immunization. However, it must not be given to pregnant women. If a pregnant woman is exposed to German measles she will continue to be given gamma globulin in an effort to prevent it. The German measles vaccine is not given to pregnant women because it is not known to what extent infection of the fetus with attenuated virus might take place. Therefore, routine immunization of adolescent girls and adult women should not be undertaken because of the danger of inadvertently administering vaccine before pregnancy is evident. Other contraindications to its use are sensitivity to chicken or duck (including eggs and feathers) and the antibiotic neomycin.

The German measles vaccine is composed of a live virus which has been weakened.

3. German Measles and Mumps Vaccine Combined. This vaccine is for simultaneous immunization against rubella and mumps for children age one to puberty. The only advantage is that of eliminating one injection. Many physicians, including myself, have not adopted the routine use of this combined vaccine (see (2) and (6) of this section).

4. Influenza Virus Vaccine. Annual influenza immunization is not recommended for all children. I recommend it for those children who have recurrent illness, who have asthma, who have congenital malformations, or those with chronic disease states such as rheumatic heart disease or diabetes.

The Public Health Service Advisory Committee on Immunization Practices has issued the following recommendations regarding dosage: Children ten years of age and older, two doses with an interval of two months between the doses. Children six to ten years of age, two doses with an interval of two months between the doses. Children three months to six years of age, three doses with an interval of one to two weeks between the first and second dose and an interval of about two months between the second and third dose.

In using the influenza virus vaccine, the first dose should be completed by early December. It is important that immunization be carried out before influenza occurs in the immediate area because there is a two week interval between injections and maximal development of protection. A single dose of vaccine can afford some protection, but is not recommended. The formula of the influenza virus vaccine is changed from time to time with the addition of new strains that prove to be clinically significant.

5. Measles Vaccine. The purpose of the measles vaccine is to prevent severe complications of measles, namely encephalitis and bronchopneumonia. The measles vaccine should be administered as soon as possible after one year old. The baby must be at least this old for proper immunity to develop. In high risk situations the vaccine may be given as early as nine months. Even after exposure to an active case of measles, the vaccine will still provide some protection if it is given within the first twenty-four to forty-eight hours. The measles vaccine provides permanent lifetime immunity. No boosters are necessary. Children immunized will develop a mild case of measles. However, they are non-contagious since the virus has been weakened. The most frequent symptom is a fever of 101 to 102 degrees. A few children may develop a fever of 103 to 104 degrees or a typical measles rash that starts on the face and progresses toward the feet. Even if these side effects occur, the patient will not act particularly sick. The advantages of the vaccine far outweigh any reactions to it. The simultaneous administration of gamma globulin as originally recommended is no longer indicated,

190

as so few children developed side effects. It is possible that a few individual children will not receive one hundred per cent protection from the vaccine, but this is a rarity. An actual case of measles, in spite of having received the vaccine should have no meaning to the parents as complications are still prevented.

The American Academy of Pediatrics has recommended that the killed measles vaccine no longer be used and that the attentuated measles vaccine be given as soon as possible to children who may have only received the killed type of vaccine. Any child who has underlying illness, or who receives forms of therapy that may render it inadvisable to administer live measles vaccine should be given gamma globulin for protection on exposure to measles. This is necessary with each exposure, since gamma globulin only affords temporary protection.

Contraindications to the live measles vaccine are egg sensitivity, recent administration of gamma globulin, pregnancy, leukemia, and current therapy with cortisone (steroids).

6. Mumps. The mumps vaccine may be used in children older than one year and is especially recommended for all males in pre-adolescent or older age groups who have not had mumps, either on one or both sides. However, in view of the usually mild nature of mumps the vaccine should be given only after all other routine immunizations of higher priority are completed. Thus, the mumps vaccine is the last one given in my opinion.

Evidence indicates that the vaccine will not offer protection when given after exposure to natural mumps.

The mumps vaccine is composed of a live virus which has been weakened. Contraindications to its use are sensitivity to eggs, chicken, chicken feathers, and the antibiotic neomycin, in addition to gamma globulin deficiency and patients receiving cortisone. The mumps vaccine is a one visit single dose injection. There are no significant clinical side effects.

7. Polio—Oral (Trivalent—Types I, II, III Combined). The oral polio vaccine is a modified live virus. Immunization against poliomyelitis with the oral vaccine has proven to be more effective than with the killed virus (Salk) vaccine. Therefore, the oral polio vaccine should be used exclusively. For *infants*, the American Academy of Pediatrics recommends three doses of oral vaccine.

The oral vaccine is administered at least a month apart. A booster or fourth dosage is given a year later. This completes the primary series.

A different recommendation was made by the special advisory committee on all poliomyelitis vaccine to the Surgeon General of the United States Public Health Service. This recommendation consists of two doses of trivalent vaccine at eight week intervals for infants and a booster third dose at the end of the first year of life. The recommendation by the American Academy of Pediatrics provides a slightly higher percentage of protection, but, the best course of action is to follow your physician's preference and get immunized.

For *school age* and *older* children, the American Academy of Pediatrics and the Surgeon General recommend two doses at six to eight week intervals. If one's past history of immunization against poliomyelitis is unknown or uncertain, or consists of the injectable form only, or only possibly one type (monovalent oral polio vaccine), two doses of trivalent vaccine (types one, two and three) combined in a single dose at intervals of no less than eight weeks are indicated. An additional booster dose of trivalent vaccine may be given to those of unusual risks such as persons living in epidemic areas. On entering elementary school all children who have completed the primary series should probably be given a single follow-up trivalent oral polio booster, according to the American Academy of Pediatrics. However, the Public Health Service Advisory Committee does not recommend routine booster doses. Follow your physician's advice.

The American Academy of Pediatrics recommends that polio vaccine not be administered at the same time the measles vaccine is administered. The Surgeon General's Committee does not consider the following conditions as contraindications to oral polio administration: tonsillectomy, tooth extraction, pregnancy, pencillin allergy, therapy with steroids (cortisone), low gamma globulin, smallpox vaccination, and DPT inoculations.

8. Rabies Vaccine.   (See Rabies.)

9. Rocky Mountain Spotted Fever (RMSF).   Two vaccines are available for protection against Rocky Mountain spotted fever. Protection against this disease is not recommended in the United States. Injections must be repeated each year. This vaccine is of no value in preventing Rocky Mountain spotted fever after the bite of an infected tick.

10. Smallpox. A vaccine containing the virus of cowpox is used to provide protection against smallpox. The smallpox vaccination should be given before eighteen months of age as it is less apt to make the baby sick when administered early in life. The site of vaccination usually is on the left arm in a skin fold where it will be less noticeable. The vaccinated area will become red, raised, filled with clear fluid, filled with pus, form a scab, fall off and leave a scar. The entire reaction will take approximately three weeks. No baths should be given the day of the vaccination. Thereafter, baths may be given. No guard, shield, or bandaid should be placed over the vaccination. However, shirts with sleeves may be worn. Sometimes the site of the vaccination will become quite red around its edges. If so, wipe around the vaccination with alcohol three or four times a day. Occasionally, the child will accidentally knock the scab completely off, leaving an ulcerated area oozing pus. Nothing special need be done as a scab will reform. The vaccination will still be successful. During the height of the reaction the baby is entitled to run a 103 to 104 degree fever. The usual fever medication is indicated. (See Aspirin, Tempra, Tylenol.) Children are usually not as sick as most parents fear.

If parents see the vaccination spreading from the original site, they should call their child's physician immediately. Spread from the original site may cause a serious generalized vaccination reaction. Contraindications to smallpox vaccination are the presence of smallpox, eczema, burns, and hypogammaglobulinemia, either in the patient or household contacts.

Occasionally vaccinations do not take. This does not mean the child is immune. The vaccination material might have lost its effectiveness upon exposure to extreme heat, or the agent used to clean the skin might not have completely evaporated. If the first vaccination is not successful, it should be repeated.

Re-vaccination is recommended every five to seven years. When a person is re-vaccinated, the stages through which it passes and the length of time necessary will be greatly shortened since some previously developed immunity will still be present.

11. Tuberculosis (BCG-Bacillus of Calmettea Guerin). (See Tuberculosis.)

12. Typhoid. Typhoid injections are not routinely recommended in the United States. They should be considered if a person is going to travel in a country where typhoid fever is a common occurrence or if an epidemic occurs. Typhoid immunizations are given once a week for three weeks. Boosters or "recall" injections are necessary every two to three years. A severe reaction consisting of fever and generalized aches and pains is not uncommon for a few days. These symptoms are best controlled with aspirin and tempra or tylenol and rest.

13. Typhus.   A vaccine is available against typhus but is not recommended in the United States. It has been useful in exposed laboratory workers. Two injections are given at intervals of ten to fourteen days. Booster injections should be given at the beginning and in the middle of the typhus season.

14. Yellow Fever.   Immunization against yellow fever is only practical if you are travelling to an area in which it is common. Yellow fever immunization is good for ten years. It is available in the United States only at special United States Public Health Centers by appointment. Call your local Health Department to find the one nearest you.

IMPETIGO (COMMONLY MISPRONOUNCED "INFANTIGO")

Impetigo is a superficial infection of the skin that is extremely common in the warmer climates.

A. Signs and Symptoms.   Impetigo appears as small boils and blisters with crusts. Small ulcerated areas occur underneath the crusts. Impetigo is most commonly found on the extremities, but can occur anywhere. Autoinoculation, secondary to itching, is common and, thus, impetigo spreads rapidly. No special laboratory studies are necessary as the clinical picture is characteristic.

B. Etiology (Cause).   Almost any bacteria may cause impetigo, but the streptococcus and the staphlococcus are extremely common offenders.

C. Treatment.   Impetigo may be treated by the child's parents without consulting their physician. Scrub the lesions with a hand brush hard enough to remove any crusts four times a day. Use Phisohex soap which inhibits the growth of bacteria. After each scrubbing apply an antibiotic ointment. Many are available in the drugstore without a prescription. Ask your pharmacist which one he recommends. If the child does not improve within a few days or if new lesions are appearing, he should be seen by his physician, since systemic antibiotic may be necessary in addition to the local measures. I am always pleased at how rapidly healing occurs.

D. Incubation Period.   A few days.

E. Period of Communicability.   Impetigo is communicable until healing occurs. It is spread by direct contact.

F. School Attendance.   School attendance should not be permitted until the sores are healed or adequate treatment is started.

G. Prevention.   The best prevention is personal hygiene.

H. Complications.   Since the streptococcus is a common cause of impetigo, rheumatic heart disease and nephritis are possible complications. These complications are preventable, however, by early and adequate treatment. In the Negro race increased areas of pigmentation frequently occur around the lesions without early treatment.

INFECTIOUS MONONUCLEOSIS

Teenagers may know this disease as the "kissing disease" because it is thought to be spread this way.

A. Signs and Symptoms.   The commonest signs are large swollen glands in the neck or elsewhere, an enlarged spleen, a flat red skin rash, jaundice (yellowness), fever, and extreme tiredness. Infectious mononucleosis may also cause headache, weight loss, dehydration, abdominal pain, and chest pain. The disease is characterized by remissions and exacerbations. A rapid screening blood test is available for use in your physician's office. The diagnosis is confirmed by a specific blood test called the "heterophile."

B. Etiology (Cause).   Probably a virus.

C. Treatment.   The treatment of choice is limitation of activity, combined with as much rest as possible. Antibiotic is of no value unless secondary infection occurs. Supportive measures, including fluids directly into a vein, strict bed rest, and prevention of anemia, may be necessary if the patient becomes dehydrated or extremely weak. The outlook for complete recovery is good even when the patient is acutely ill. Many patients develop this disease and recover spontaneously, never knowing they had it.

D. Incubation Period.   Four to fourteen days.

E. Period of Communicability.   Unknown. Infectious mononucleosis is of low grade contagion.

F. School Attendance.   School attendance is permissible providing the patient does not become overly tired.

G. Prevention.   There is no known prevention.

H. Complications.   Involvement of the liver causing marked jaundice (yellowness) may lead to permanent liver impairment, but only under the rarest of circumstances.

INFLUENZA, GRIPPE, VIREMIA, FLU

These four names are frequently used to refer to the same illness. The symptoms are the familiar ones of:

1. Fever.
2. Chills.
3. Headache.
4. Muscle and joint pains.
5. Tiredness.
6. Nausea.
7. Vomiting.
8. Diarrhea.

If the breathing passages are the site of infection, the following are frequent complaints:

(a) Stuffy and runny nose.
(b) Sore throat.
(c) Coughing.
(d) Raising of phlegm.
(e) Chest discomfort.

Influenza is caused by a number of different viruses. These viruses are present more or less constantly in the population and tend to break out from time to time in a flurry of cases. Fortunately, these viral infections are more uncomfortable than they are dangerous. Antibiotic is of no value. Symptomatic treatment will usually tide the patient over until his natural recovery takes place. Specific suggestions are given under the treatment of the common cold. These infections notoriously sap the strength of the patient for several weeks after the acute stage has subsided. Recurrences are common, since the immunity acquired is fleeting. There is no effective way to immunize people against these infections except for certain forms of influenza. (See Immunizations.)

196

INGROWN NAIL

Ingrown toenails and fingernails may be prevented by cutting the nails straight across without rounding them. Ingrown nails are painful and secondary infection is common. Consult your physician. Antibiotic therapy to counteract the infection is not sufficient in most cases. The nail must usually be removed.

INSECT BITES

Insect bites vary in size and shape from huge hives to small red bumps. The swelling and redness is caused by an allergic reaction in the skin. A tiny hole may be noticeable in the center of the bump. In uncomplicated cases, start treatment without consulting your doctor. Antihistamine is used to control the swelling. Triaminic syrup is available in the drugstore without a prescription. See Colds —Treatment for the recommended dosage. Secondary infection (impetigo) commonly occurs because bug bites itch and children scratch. This may be controlled by applying Caladryl (calamine) lotion on a when-necessary basis. It is available in the drugstore without a prescription. Treatment of superficial infection consists of Phisohex scrubs, followed by local antibiotic ointment. Rarely is systemic antibiotic necessary. (See Impetigo.)

Bug repellents such as "612" or "Off," available as a spray, liquid or stick, are valuable in decreasing the number of bites from certain insects such as mosquitoes. They are available over the counter and are safe for use at any age.

An allergic reaction from the bite of stinging insects may progress far enough to cause swelling of the airway and difficulty in breathing. The signs and symptoms of croup may develop. (See Croup.) Call your physician immediately. Potent medication is necessary to counteract the allergic reaction.

There are more deaths in the United States each year from stinging insect bites than anyone imagines. Recently fifty deaths were reported in one state. The principal offenders are the yellow jacket, bee, wasp, and hornet, which belong to the order hymenoptera. These insects are widely distributed throughout the United States. Certain drugs given immediately to hypersensitive patients following the insect sting or bite may prove lifesaving. For emergencies, Center Laboratories has made available an easy-to-carry kit containing:

1. Adrenalin.
2. A tourniquet to limit spread of venom.
3. Ephedrine Sulfate Tablets.
4. Antihistamine.
5. Sterile alcohol pad.
6. Complete instructions for effective use.

This kit is available at your local drugstore by prescription. It is designed for pocket or purse. It is especially recommended for:

1. Hymenoptera sensitive persons.
2. Campers.
3. Outdoorsmen and sportsmen.
4. Farmers.
5. Gardeners.

Desensitization shots to stinging insects are mandatory if a severe allergic reaction has ever occurred. (See Asthma and the Allergic Patient.) Common sense would also dictate avoiding such places as national parks, camp sites and other areas where stinging insects are more common.

INTERTRIGO

Intertrigo is an irritation of the skin that occurs when two moist surfaces rub against each other. The skin becomes bright red and appears raw. It frequently appears in the folds of the skin around the neck, behind the ears and in the groin. Intertrigo is more common in infants who sweat a lot or are obese. Treatment consists of frequent baths and dusting powder. Improvement should be rapid; if not, consult your physician.

INTESTINAL OBSTRUCTION

Intestinal obstruction means blockage has occurred in the stomach or intestines that interferes with the passage of food or waste material. The signs and symptoms all of which are not always present, include:

1. Excessive mucous that accumulates in the infant's throat.
2. Vomiting.
3. Distention of the abdomen (belly).

4. Absent or decreased stools.
5. Paroxysms of pain or crying.
6. Loss of weight.
7. Dehydration with associated fever.

Special X rays in which barium is used as a contrast medium helps the physician arrive at a specific diagnosis.

The usual causes of intestinal obstruction in children are defined below. With the exception of pyloric stenosis, which is discussed in detail, most of these conditions are extremely rare. Surgery is the treatment of choice in most cases. The outlook for survival depends upon a number of factors such as the baby's weight, general condition, the presence of other abnormalities, and how early the diagnosis is made.

1. Anular Pancreas. A ring of pancreatic tissue encircles part of the small intestine, thereby obstructing the normal route through the digestive tract.

2. Congenital Megacolon (Hirschsprung's Disease). There is a deficiency in the nervous inervation of the rectum. The stools are passed out of the rectum with difficulty. The lower part of the intestine (colon) becomes enlarged in an attempt to force the stools out.

3. Esophageal Atresia. Atresia is the congenital absence of a passage. The upper end of the esophagus ends in a blind pouch. The upper end of the lower esophagus forms a connection between the stomach and trachea (airway) in ninety per cent of the cases. The diagnosis is easily established. A soft rubber tube cannot be passed into the stomach.

4. Imperforate Anus. There is an absence of the normal opening between the buttocks that allows stool to pass to the outside.

5. Incarcerated Inguinal Hernia. A portion of the bowel becomes caught in the sac of the hernia resulting in obstruction to the blood supply and possibly death of the bowel. (See Hernia (Rupture.)

6. Intestinal Atresia. One end of the intestine ends in a blind pouch. It is not continuous with the rest of the intestine.

7. Intussusception. One part of the intestine telescopes into another part.

8. Malrotation.   Twisting of the intestine occurs because it is not located in its normal position.

9. Meconium Illeus.   This is a mechanical obstruction due to impacted sticky meconium that occasionally occurs in cystic fibrosis. (See Cystic Fibrosis.)

10. Pyloric Stenosis.   The opening between the stomach and the first part of the intestine is obstructed by an overly well developed muscle. Pyloric stenosis is the commonest obstruction found in infants. It is more common in males by a five to one ratio. Its unique symptoms allow the physician to readily establish the diagnosis.

The symptoms usually begin in the second or third week of life; rarely as late as the second month. There is projectile vomiting which is forceful in nature. The vomitus will shoot out. At times it will come out of the nose. It does not contain bile, which is green in color, since the obstruction is at the end of the stomach. Bile enters into the first part of the intestine. Constipation becomes progressively worse until there are no stools, since less food is getting beyond the stomach. Weight loss and dehydration finally occur.

On physical examination your physician may be able to feel an olive-sized pyloric mass which represents the over-developed muscle. When indicated, the diagnosis may be confirmed by X-ray studies. A complete cure is afforded by cutting the over-developed muscle fibers. After surgery the infant may be fed almost immediately upon awakening. Medical treatment without surgery is not acceptable.

11. Volvulus.   Twisting of the intestine occurs which interferes with the normal blood supply. If the blood supply is interfered with long enough, the intestine may die.

K

KNOCK KNEES

Knock knees are commonly seen in children three and four years of age. They are perfectly normal at this time. In most cases no treatment is necessary. The condition is self-limited and corrects itself as the child grows. If knock knees are marked, basic underlying causes such as rickets or injury should be considered. An X ray is advisable under these circumstances.

L

LARYNGITIS

The larynx is an area deep in the back of the throat where the vocal chords are located. Infection involving the larynx is called laryngitis.

A. Signs and Symptoms. Acute laryngitis is usually precipitated by a cold. In mild cases which last for only a few days, there is hoarseness, fever and a general feeling of tiredness. There is no difficulty in breathing. In severe cases, the disease progresses after a few days to the point where the child may completely lose his voice. The temperature may rise to 103 or 105 degrees. At this stage difficulty in breathing is usually present. The signs and symptoms of respiratory distress are sucking in, in the neck, between the ribs, under the rib cage and moving in and out of the nose as the child breathes.

B. Etiology (Cause). Laryngitis can be either a viral or bacterial infection.

C. Treatment. Your physician should be consulted in most cases because there usually is some involvement of adjacent tissues. Thus, the disease may progress into epiglottitis or croup. (See Epiglottitis, Croup.) Specific antibiotic therapy is indicated when laryngitis is bacterial in origin. When laryngitis is viral in origin antibiotic is of no value. Antihistamine helps reduce the swelling and thus eliminates some of the hoarseness. Occasionally, gargling with S.T.37 or some such similar preparation may be of value. S.T.37 is available in the drugstore without a prescription, and directions for its use are on the package. One teaspoon of whiskey mixed with one tablespoon of honey is an old-fashioned remedy which may relieve some of the local symptoms. A vaporizer may be extremely helpful. Rest is always important.

LARYNGOMALACIA (CONGENITAL LARYNGEAL STRIDOR)

In laryngomalacia the vocal chords are more relaxed than normal and the epiglottis, which is the little lump that sticks up in the back of the throat when saying "ah" may be floppy. The major symptom is the presence of stridor (crowing sound) when the child breathes in, sometimes associated with periods of blueness of the lips (cyanosis). The condition is apparently connected in some way with calcium metabolism. No special examinations are necessary unless the stridor is unusually severe. Children will outgrow laryngomalacia between sixteen and twenty-four months of age. There is no specific treatment and special care is not necessary.

LEAD POISONING

Since the widespread use of lead-free paints, lead poisoning is no longer a common problem. Previously children frequently developed chronic lead poisoning from chewing on window sills which were covered with paint containing lead. Lead poisoning may also occur from the inhalation of fumes from burning battery casings.

The signs and symptoms may be divided into those affecting:

1. The *gastrointestinal tract*—
     (a) persistent vomiting;
     (b) constipation;
     (c) abdominal pain.
2. The *central nervous system*—
     (a) visual disturbance;
     (b) delirium;
     (c) convulsions.
3. The *blood*—
     (a) secondary anemia.

Occasionally, a black line is found in the gums called a lead line. The incidence is highest from one to three years of age. The diagnosis is proven by determining the amount of lead in the urine. Certain changes also occur in the red blood cells which may be seen when a complete blood count is done. X rays may reveal an increased density at the growing ends of the long bones of the body.

The treatment consists of a diet high in calcium and phosphorus, with large amounts of vitamin D. Two very good drugs are available for the treatment of acute lead poisoning. The results of treatment are excellent. In chronic lead poisoning deleading with specific drugs such as BAL or EDTA is dangerous. The body probably should be left alone to excrete the lead gradually over a long period of time.

LEUKEMIA

Leukemia is a malignancy of the blood in which the white blood cells proliferate profusely. It is an extremely rare disease that occurs most frequently between the ages of two and five. Leukemia seems more prevalent than it is because of the publicity that the affected children receive in the local newspapers.

The signs and symptoms are primarily due to infiltration of the body by malignant cells. There is interference with normal blood production. The signs and symptoms include:

1. Bone and joint pain.
2. Enlarged liver.
3. Enlarged lymph glands.
4. Enlarged spleen.
5. Easy bruising.
6. Fatigue.
7. Fever.
8. Little areas of hemorrhage under the skin.
9. Loss of appetite.
10. Reduced resistance to infection.
11. Weight loss.

A routine blood count will rule this disease out. If the blood count is abnormal the diagnosis is confirmed by examining the bone marrow where the white blood cells are produced. Obtaining bone marrow is not difficult or painful for the child and doesn't require hospitalization.

Many physicians feel that leukemia is caused by a virus. If this is so, eventually a vaccine will be developed to prevent it.

The treatment of choice depends upon the specific type of leukemia present which is determined by what type of white blood cells are involved. Eight drugs are now available that have produced remissions and the therapeutic picture is guardedly optimistic. New treatment regimens continue to increase the remission rate of acute childhood leukemia. During remissions the patient is perfectly well and may be allowed complete activity. However, there is no cure for leukemia. The outlook is best for lymphacytic leukemia where patients who survive five years have a one-in-four chance of still being in complete remission at ten years. Total body irradiation and transplantation of bone marrow has been tried. The results are still experimental. A new process has been developed called extra-corporeal irradiation of the blood. The whole process is conducted in a closed system employing a plastic tube pipeline which runs from one of the patient's arteries, in and out of a dome-like ir-radiator near the patient's bedside and back into the body through a vein.

This type of research gives us added hope that in time we may come to control and conquer this dread disease.

LICE (PEDICULOSIS)

Pediculosis means the patient is infested with lice.

A. Signs and Symptoms.   The outstanding symptom is severe itching. The scratching is intense enough to abrade the skin, causing a discharge of fluid which forms crusts and mats the hair together. The nits or eggs are found in the hair.

B. Etiology (Cause).   A louse. This is a general name for various parasitic insects.

C. Treatment.   A five to ten per cent solution of DDT and talcum is rubbed into the scalp and is allowed to remain for twenty-four hours. The hair is then washed. The treatment is repeated two weeks later to kill any newly hatched lice.

D. Period of Communicability.   Lice are spread directly by contact and indirectly by clothing, and are, therefore, communicable until killed.

E. School Attendance.   Treatment must be completed before the patient returns to school.

F. Preventive Measures.   Personal hygiene prevents lice.

LIMPING

Limping is a common complaint that physicians who take care of children are faced with almost daily. Parents unfortunately think of the worst possible diagnoses. Limping is generally due to an un-observed fall that causes bleeding under the periostium, which covers the bone. Usually there are no abnormal findings on physical or X-ray examination. However, if an X ray were taken three weeks later it would confirm the diagnosis because the calcium in the blood under the periostium would be visible. Therefore, most doctors faced with the problem of limping do not take an X ray unless the child fails to recover in three to four weeks, providing the child's physical examination is normal. I suggest no specific studies or treatment. Be patient. However, if the limping does not disappear within three to four weeks, X rays should be ordered.

If the child's physical examination is not normal, a complete workup, including laboratory studies and X rays, is indicated.

M

MEASLES (RUBELLA)

It is not difficult for parents to make the diagnosis of this childhood disease. Measles is a systemic disease that involves the whole body. It is not confined to the skin just because a rash is present.

A. Signs and Symptoms.   Measles begins with a cold. The eyes become red. This is called conjunctivitis (pink eye). The fever gradually increases and a rash appears about the fourth day when the fever is usually 103 degrees, or more. The rash is flat and red. *It starts on the face and progresses toward the feet.* The rash gradually becomes larger and may coalesce with other spots, so it may look as if the entire skin is covered. The day before the rash breaks out there are Koplik spots inside the mouth by the lower molar teeth. These are white patches of tissue surrounded by small red areas. Parents need not look for them, as sometimes they are even difficult for your doctor to recognize. Cough is a very common symptom that usually becomes progressively worse for at least a few days. As the child improves, the rash will disappear in the order in which it appeared.

B. Etiology (Cause).   Measles is a viral infection.

C. Treatment.   I believe that it is best for your physician to see your child at least once during the course of this illness because many children become quite ill. Unfortunately, there is no specific treatment since antibiotic therapy is of no value in a viral infection. However, antibiotic is effective if secondary invasion by bacteria occurs, causing complications such as infected ears. Aspirin with tempra or tylenol are given to control the fever. (See Aspirin, Tempra, Tylenol.) For mild coughs use a cough medication which is available in the drugstore without a prescription. Ask your pharmacist to recommend one to you along with the proper dosage. If the cough should be deep and sound severe, or is not relieved by the usual cough medication, stronger cough preparations are available by prescription. The patient's room need not be kept dark. Television may be permitted as long as the child doesn't complain about his eyes. Nothing will make the rash come out. The average child without complications will be sick for one week, but may require another week to recuperate and gain strength.

D. Incubation. The incubation period is ten to twelve days.

E. Period of Communicability. Measles is communicable four days before the rash appears to five days after the rash is present.

F. School Attendance. Any child with measles should be isolated at home for at least seven days following the appearance of the rash. Other children in the family may attend school, but are to be observed carefully for the first sign of illness, at which time they are to remain home.

G. Prevention. Measles no longer needs to be a serious childhood illness with complications since it is now a preventable disease. More than twenty-five million children have now received the measles vaccine in the United States. Experts estimate that the disease eradication campaign has prevented about twenty-five thousand cases of measles encephalitis and ten thousand cases of mental retardation. (See Immunizations.)

H. Complications. Complications should be minor with adequate prevention. The serious complications of pneumonia and encephalitis leading to possible brain damage may be avoided by proper immunization. These complications are serious because there is no specific therapy for them. (See Pneumonia and Encephalitis.) Unfortunately, measles is still a leading cause of death in children throughout the developing nations. Despite measles becoming a preventable illness the National Communicable Disease Center estimates that seven million children remain susceptible. Only through constant vigilance and immunization of all children can the incidence of measles and its complications be kept to a minimum.

MENINGITIS

Meningitis is a serious infection involving the central nervous system. Before the advent of antibiotic therapy, it was a frequent complication of other disease conditions. *If meningitis is suspected, your physician should be called immediately.*

A. Signs and Symptoms.   The following signs and symptoms may be present:

1. Stiff neck.
2. Fever.
3. Headache.
4. Vomiting.
5. Increased muscle tone.
6. Overactive reflexes.
7. Abnormal reflexes.
8. Twitching.
9. Convulsions.
10. Drowsiness.

The classical sign which is *not always present* early in the illness is a *stiff neck*. The child will be unable to touch his chin to the upper part of his chest. Sometimes unexplained high fever in a very small child is the only symptom. The diagnosis is most difficult to establish, even with a thorough history and physical examination. For this reason, if your physician suspects meningitis he must do a lumbar puncture. A lumbar puncture (spinal tap) is far less dangerous than an undiagnosed case of meningitis. Under sterile conditions with local anesthesia a needle is placed between the lower vertebra in the small of the back. Fluid is then withdrawn from the spinal canal and sent to the laboratory for analysis. This is the same procedure frequently used in obstetrics for anesthesia, except that after the spinal fluid is withdrawn an anesthetic agent is used to replace it. Certain changes occur in the spinal fluid that are diagnostic of meningitis.

B. Etiology (Cause).   Meningitis is caused by specific bacteria and different kinds of viruses. The commonest bacteria involved are the pneumococcus, meningococcus and hemophilus influenzae.

C. Treatment.   All diagnostic and therapeutic measures must be carried out as rapidly as possible. A single hour's delay may lessen the chance of recovery. The treatment depends upon the cause. Triple antibiotic therapy is frequently started until the specific organism is isolated, at which time one or more of the antibiotics may be stopped. Sensitivity tests are performed in the laboratory to determine what antibiotic the causative organism will respond to best. These tests are correlated with the patient's clinical response. Antibiotic therapy is usually started directly into the patient's veins until there is marked improvement. Therapy is continued for a minimum of one to three weeks depending upon the bacteria isolated. Other measures include the maintenance of proper fluids, prevention of anemia by giving blood if necessary, control of headache, and sedation if convulsions occur. An oxygen tent may be necessary in the critically ill. Since no physician can predict the outcome, all known measures of treatment are used. I have seen many children critically ill in a coma survive and attain a complete recovery without complications.

Infection in the nervous system caused by a virus is called asceptic meningitis. Antibiotic therapy is of no value. However, all other measures are indicated.

D. Incubation Period.   The incubation period depends on the child's ability to fight a local infection. Therefore, it cannot be categorically stated except for meningococcal meningitis, where it may be as short as twenty-four hours.

E. Period of Communicability.   Only meningococcal meningitis is highly contagious. (See Prevention below.) As a matter of fact, most hospital cases of meningitis do not need to be isolated.

F. School Attendance.   The patient may go back to school when he is completely well, as determined by his physician.

G. Prevention.   Since meningitis is often a complication of other infections such as ear infections, sinus infections, or pussy lesions of the head and scalp, which may constitute the portal of entry, adequate and early treatment of all illness is necessary. One type of meningitis is frequently preceded or accompanied by a cold. If your child does not recover from a cold within a few days, he should be checked. *Upon exposure to meningococcal meningitis,* *sulfa must be taken for one week to prevent this highly contagious disease.* If the person exposed is allergic to sulfa, penicillin may be substituted. *The contacts include the parents, relatives, friends who have stopped by the house, the teacher, and all children in the same classroom in school.* No medication can prevent any other form of meningitis. *Before calling your physician find out what kind of meningitis your child was exposed to.*

H. Complications. With early diagnosis and treatment, complications are rare. Complications are common when treatment has been started late in the course of the illness. They include deafness, blindness, hydrocephalus, pneumonia, arthritis, involvement of the heart, paralysis, mental retardation, shock, and a collection of fluid underneath the covering of the brain, called a subdural hematoma. All collections of fluid must be surgically drained.

MOLES

Moles are areas of increased pigmentation found in the skin. They vary in size and shape—some are pinpoint in nature and others may be several inches long. Most moles are harmless and require no treatment. However, if a mole increases rapidly in size, is dark in color like a black telephone cord, or is located in an area where irritation and injury is common, it should be surgically excised. This can usually be done in your physician's office. The specimen is then sent to a pathologist who will examine it under the microscope. A pathologist is a medical doctor who has specialized in studying the changes which are caused by disease. Practically no moles are malignant in children, but certain types of moles may become malignant with advanced age. By surgically removing moles which are changing in character, serious problems are prevented.

MONGOLISM

A Mongoloid baby has a peculiar looking appearance that is associated with some degree of mental retardation. He is born with some of the following characteristics: slanted eyes, high cheek bones, a flat nose, a short and inward curved fifth finger, and poor muscle tone. Since many family characteristics such as high cheek bones and slanted eyes are inherited, parents must be careful not to confuse them with those of Mongolism. In addition, congenital heart disease is found more frequently associated with Mongolism than would be normally expected.

Mongolism is caused by an abnormal chromosome and, therefore, heredity is the most important factor. *From a genetic standpoint further pregnancies should be avoided if the parents already have one Mongoloid child.* Age of the expectant mother and sex of the infant are other factors. When an older woman conceives, Mongolism is more apt to occur. The incidence is slightly higher in males.

No physician can predict how bright a Mongoloid baby will be. Some Mongoloid children are capable of taking care of their daily needs, but are not smart enough to react to emergencies. A few may be educated in special schools. However, the vast majority are probably not capable of taking care of themselves. Certainly it is safe to say that a Mongoloid child will not meet the usual standards of development. Therefore, providing special care in a nursing home for retarded children or in a state institution should be seriously considered. Some physicians believe this should be done immediately after birth. They feel that if the baby does not go home with the parents there is less likelihood of developing strong emotional ties that might be difficult to break as the baby grows older.

Other physicians believe that it is better for the parents to care for their Mongoloid baby at home until they see that the baby is affecting other members of the family, or that they are not capable of dealing with the child on an everyday basis. From a practical standpoint there is such a long waiting list for admission to state institutions that the affected child is frequently not admitted until three to five years of age. Therefore, application should be made as soon as a decision has been reached. I cannot tell parents what to do. This is a decision for parents to make on an individual basis after reviewing all aspects of the problem. They must, however, take into consideration their own feelings. I believe that they should discuss their feelings with a clinical psychologist or psychiatrist. Too often decisions are made for a different reason than the parents are willing to admit to themselves.

The parents of a Mongoloid baby have no legitimate reason to feel guilty. They should not make martyrs of themselves for the rest of their lives. A short life expectancy for the child is not unusual.

210

Mongoloid babies frequently succumb early in life to congenital heart disease and severe infections.

MOTION SICKNESS

Motion sickness from riding in an automobile, boat or airplane will often induce vomiting in children. If this is a recurrent problem, medication such as Dramamine given approximately one hour prior to traveling will be helpful. It is available in the drugstore without a prescription. For children six to eight years of age, the dose is one to two teaspoons two or three times a day. For children eight to twelve years of age, the dose is two to four teaspoons two or three times a day. If oral medication cannot be retained, suppositories for rectal administration are available. These suppositories contain the equivalent of eight teaspoons of liquid Dramamine. Therefore, if the parents want to give the equivalent of two teaspoons of the liquid, one-quarter of a suppository would be required.

MUMPS

Mumps is an infection involving the salivary glands found at the angle of the jaw and in the floor of the mouth. It is not necessary to see your doctor in most cases. If in doubt, the diagnosis can often be confirmed by telephone. Both sides of the neck are usually involved, but one side may be involved to a much lesser degree so that it is not obvious to you, the parent. However, it is possible for mumps to involve only one side. Mumps is a mild childhood disease. It is possible to contract the disease more than once.

A. Signs and Symptoms.   A painful swelling appears at the angle of the jaw and in front of the ear. The ear lobe appears to be in the center of the swelling. Fever between 101 and 102 degrees is usually present. Citrus fruit as well as hard chewing movements may make the pain worse.

Mumps must be distinguished from swollen infected glands that may also occur in the neck. Swollen infected glands usually occur lower in the neck and have a harder feel. Swollen glands from mumps are more gelatinous to touch. If the case is not clear cut, the child should be seen by his physician. If the patient develops high fever, abdominal pain, swelling of the testicles or any symptoms involving the nervous system, such as irritability and drowsiness, he should also be seen by his physician.

B. Etiology (Cause).   Mumps is a viral infection.

C. Treatment.   Adequate treatment consists of rest, fluids and aspirin with tempra or tylenol for pain and fever. Antibiotic is of no value.

D. Incubation.   The incubation period is twelve to twenty-six days, more commonly eighteen.

E. Period of Communicability.   Mumps is communicable from a few days prior to the onset of symptoms, until the swelling disappears.

F. School Attendance.   School should not be attended until the swelling completely disappears. Other children in the family may attend school until they develop the first signs and symptoms of mumps.

G. Prevention.   (See Immunizations.)

H. Complications.   The virus of mumps may spread to the testicles, central nervous system and pancreas. Swelling of the testicles with associated pain is extremely rare, particularly when one considers that this is a common childhood illness. The treatment consists of strict bed rest and support for the testicles. Although sterility can result this seems to me to be more of a theoretical possibility than a practical problem. The symptoms of the mumps virus invading the central nervous system are the same as those of encephalitis and meningitis. (See Encephalitis and Meningitis.) This complication is not common and when it does occur the resulting illness is mild so that hospitalization is often not necessary. If the virus invades the pancreas located in the belly, abdominal pain and vomiting may result. There is no specific treatment for these complications, but general measures including rest, fluids and control of pain are adequate.

N

NAIL BITING

Nail biting is common and is a sign of nervousness. Children may start biting their nails while watching a monster show on television.

Constantly reminding the child not to bite his nails is usually not successful. Putting foul tasting material on the nails does not work either. The nail biter seldom realizes what he is doing. Try to find out what is causing the tension. It usually is not a serious problem. If the scary shows on television are causing it, they should be avoided. Sometimes a mature two year old girl will do well by having a nail polishing set. Perhaps if the mother will help her daughter polish her nails, this will make her act in a more grown up fashion.

NAVEL (BELLY BUTTON)

The umbilical artery and veins run through the navel. This is how the baby is nourished by the mother in her uterus. After birth, the doctor ties and cuts the umbilical cord. The remaining stump dries up by three weeks of age and falls off, leaving the belly button. No special care of the umbilical cord is necessary while it is drying. When the cord is off a tub bath is given. Until then the infant is given a sponge bath. Excessive scar tissue sometimes builds up into a pea size mass. This is called a granuloma. It is not malignant. Treatment consists of applying silver nitrate, which cauterizes the scar tissue. This does not hurt the baby. The surrounding skin may be temporarily blackened. More than one treatment is often required.

Types of Navel. (1) *Skin Type*—If the skin extends onto the navel cord, your obstetrician is not able to cut it off. The resultant navel will be rather large with a great deal of fleshy skin that protrudes from the belly wall. This will look particularly poor while the child is young and naturally pot-bellied. As the child grows older and the abdominal cavity (belly) enlarges, this fleshy skin will become less obvious. (2) The *flat type* in which the skin is level with the abdominal wall. (3) The *depressed type* in which there is very little skin on the umbilical cord leaving a fairly marked depression.

All these types are normal and no plastic surgery is necessary.

Bleeding. Bleeding from the navel commonly occurs when the umbilical cord detaches itself spontaneously by three weeks of age, or sooner. If bleeding occurs wipe the cord off with alcohol four times a day. If the bleeding persists for more than two or

213

three days, consult your physician. Do not use a binder or bandage. Deaths in infants have been reported associated with the application of tight umbilical binders that interfere with normal breathing.

NEPHRITIS (GLOMERULONEPHRITIS, BRIGHT'S DISEASE)

Nephritis means inflammation of the kidney. Since the advent of antibiotics this disease is becoming less frequent. Your physician should be consulted in all suspected cases.

A. Signs and Symptoms.   Ten days to three weeks prior to the onset of nephritis there may be a history of an upper respiratory infection, tonsillitis, scarlet fever, or impetigo. Following this, blood is found in the urine. If enough bleeding occurs, the urine may be bloody to the naked eye. The eyes may swell, especially in the morning and the ankles are often swollen too. The blood pressure may be elevated, and if high enough headache and vomiting may occur. Congestive heart failure may occur, as demonstrated by fluid collecting in the lungs and an enlarged tender liver. The usual constitutional symptoms are mild fever, tiredness, and pallor. Various simple laboratory tests are available to determine the degree of involvement of the kidneys.

B. Etiology (Cause).   Nephritis is caused by an allergic reaction to a streptococcal infection.

C. Treatment.   In my opinion all cases should be hospitalized for a complete workup and adequate rest, which is frequently impossible for the parents to enforce at home. If a strep infection is still present, it must be completely eradicated. Penicillin is the drug of choice for all strep infections. If the child is allergic to penicillin, another antibiotic may be substituted. I recommend an injection of a long acting penicillin, called bicillin, that will last for two weeks. Some physicians may prefer to place the patient on oral penicillin for a minimum of ten days. The patient must have complete bed rest until healing of the kidneys is almost complete. This is indicated by the disappearance of the clinical signs and symptoms. The sedimentation rate, which is a nonspecific blood test that shows activity of any nature, is an excellent way of following the course of this disease. As the patient improves the sedimentation rate will return to normal. Adequate medications are available to control any com-

214

plications such as high blood pressure or heart failure. Complete healing occurs in the vast majority of cases, usually in six to eight weeks.

D. Incubation. The incubation period is ten days to three weeks following a strep infection.

E. Period of Communicability. Nephritis, per se, is not a communicable disease, but any streptococcal infection is highly contagious until treated.

F. School Attendance. The patient may return to school with the approval of his physician.

G. Prevention. Prevention is the best treatment for nephritis. It may be prevented by the early and vigorous treatment of all streptococcal infections. If your child has a cold that does not repond to conservative measures in a few days, he should be seen by his physician. A strep infection may be present without throat pain. If impetigo does not respond to conservative measures within a few days, it should be treated by your physician. All cases of scarlet fever must be seen immediately by your physician. A medical expert on streptococcal infections has recommended that any child exposed to a strep infection be given preventive penicillin therapy. This means that if a well child is exposed to a strep infection *in close quarters* such as the home, he should receive preventive penicillin. This does not apply to the school situation. Many physicians follow this procedure in their practice.

H. Complications. The most serious complications are the development of chronic nephritis and kidney failure. Some cases go on for several months before complete healing occurs. Therefore, nephritis should not be designated as chronic unless abnormal findings persist in the urine for six months or longer. Many chronic cases are mild and do not interfere with living a useful life. Human beings have much more kidney capacity than they require. Some chronic cases may finally develop uremia (kidney failure). If this occurs it usually is a slow process that takes many years, and thus it is not a problem until much later in life. Many adults with kidney failure are adequately treated over a long period of time by use of an artificial kidney on a weekly out-patient basis. An artificial kidney gets rid of the waste products that accumulate in the blood stream due to improper kidney function. The other complications of high blood pressure and heart failure have already been mentioned, and are almost an integral part of the disease. The availability of adequate therapy needs to be emphasized.

It is important that the long-term approach be used. A child with chronic nephritis should be seen by a physician at regular intervals so that all the advances of modern medicine can be used to help him.

NEPHROSIS

Nephrosis is a syndrome occurring in young children characterized by massive swelling involving the entire body. It is a chronic disease usually extending over many years noted for its spontaneous remissions and exacerbations. All new cases should be hospitalized.

The diagnosis is confirmed by laboratory studies which reveal a large amount of albumin (protein) in urine and an elevation of the blood cholesterol level. The normal amount of protein found in the blood is also decreased. The disease process is followed by the sedimentation rate which is a nonspecific test of activity.

The cause of nephrosis is not known, but it has been suggested that it may be a phase of chronic glomerulo nephritis. (See Nephritis.)

Therapy consists of very large doses of prednisone (cortisone). The goal of therapy is to return the patient to as nearly a normal state as possible, judged by both clinical and laboratory findings. In favorable cases, the patient will begin to get rid of the excessive body fluid approximately 10 to 14 days after the beginning of therapy. This is called diuresis. Many physicians at this time give additional potassium since potassium loss is characteristic of patients on cortisone. Around this time the albumin in the urine will disappear and the blood tests will begin to return to normal. Treatment with prednisone is continued every day until the sedimentation rate returns to normal in approximately three to four weeks. After this the initial dose of prednisone is gradually tapered until it is eliminated for four days. Then the patient is started on prednisone therapy for three days out of each week. At this time the patient may be discharged from the hospital.

After this the parents must test the urine for albumin at home by the use of simple test sticks made of impregnated paper. The urine should be tested just before and just after each period of cortisone administration. If after several weeks these tests show themselves to be consistently negative for albumin, the dose of cortisone may be reduced slightly while continuing the same intermittent therapy. As long as no protein appears in the urine, the dose of cortisone may be reduced every few weeks until it can be eliminated entirely. If, however, albumin reappears in the urine, the dose of cortisone must be increased until the albumin is controlled. Cortisone therapy usually has to be continued for a year or more.

The most difficult complication to deal with is that of recurrent infections because prolonged cortisone therapy lowers the body's ability to fight infection. Often preventive antibiotic is a necessity. Other complications include high blood pressure, renal failure, and gastrointestinal bleeding. With patients who are older, feelings of both the parents and the child must be dealt with. With early remission parents may have the tendency to minimize the seriousness of this illness.

NEUROBLASTOMA

Neuroblastoma is one of the few malignancies that occurs in children. The most important finding is an abdominal mass. Each time your baby has a well-baby visit, your physician will check his abdomen and feel for such a mass. If nothing else were done at each visit, I would consider this a good enough reason for monthly well-baby check-ups during the first year of life. By the time mother discovers the mass for the first time while she is bathing the baby, it is too late for much hope.

Neuroblastoma originates from special cells called neuroblasts that form a part of the adrenal gland. The diagnosis is proven by examining the malignant cells under the microscope. This is done by means of a biopsy which is the excision for diagnostic study of a piece of tissue from a living body.

There is no known cure, but survival is possible for a number of years. Hope should not be lost since spontaneous cures or remissions have been reported in the medical literature. Treatment consists of surgery, X-ray therapy and anticancer drugs.

NEWBORN BABY (INFANTS)

Shortly after your baby is born the physician of your choice will examine your baby. If any problems are anticipated by your obstetrician, he will alert your baby's physician so that he may be present at the delivery.

No feedings are given the newborn for the first twelve hours of life. Following this, glucose water is started for a period of time before the baby starts on the bottle or is breast fed.

How long should the average newborn stay in the hospital? A week was considered routine a few years ago. Now some babies go home in two days. In my opinion the baby should have the total advantage of nursery care for a minimum of three or four days.

Let us consider some of the changes that occur after birth so that we may better understand how the newborn can be colicky, overactive and just yell like mad at times in spite of what mother does. The circulation of the blood changes. The lungs which were previously not expanded, gradually expand over a period of approximately a week and not with the first cry as most people think. During the first week of life the respiratory rate is more rapid than later on and the respirations may be somewhat irregular. In the intestines the muscles are weak, which permits them to become distended with gas easily. Food moves more slowly through the gastrointestinal tract, occasionally remaining in the stomach for twice the length of time as in the adult. Yet, the bowels are emptied more rapidly. The absorption of fat is not as efficient as in the adult. Salivation is not yet adequate and there are meconium and transitional stools. Albumin may be present in the urine along with a few pus cells during the first week of life, which is not normal thereafter. The nervous system is not fully developed. A startle (moro) reflex is present. (See #19 this section.) A rooting reflex is present. When the infant smells milk he turns his head to find the source and when his cheek is touched by an object the lips are opened as if to grasp it.

Is it any wonder that some babies have a more difficult time in making these adjustments than others? An infant requires time for all his body systems to operate in unison with each other. When he makes these necessary adjustments everybody will be happy.

Most newborns are different than the preconceived image which the parents had prior to the baby's birth. The parents may have anticipated a beautiful infant with clear, smooth skin, a perfectly round head and straight legs. Some babies may come close to meeting these criteria, but not many. Let us look at the normal variations that can be expected in the vast majority of newborns.

1. Birth Marks.   Most babies, when examined carefully enough, will have flat non-elevated irregular shaped birth marks that are pink or red in color. These are called hemangiomas and are very frequently found on the eyelids, hair line and the upper lip. They gradually fade without specific treatment.

2. Blue Buttocks.   Occasionally, a well defined bluish silvery non-elevated area of pigmentation is observed, particularly over the lower back. They are prevalent in the Negro race. The pigmentation usually fades in early childhood. It is called a Mongolian blue spot, but there is absolutely no connection with such a spot and a Mongoloid baby.

3. Bowed Legs.   Since the baby was contained inside the mother's uterus for approximately nine months, the legs are often bowed, or there is a mild deviation of the foot without any bone deformity. This is the result of the fetal position. These normal variations will gradually correct themselves, especially after a baby begins to walk.

4. Breast.   Enlargement of the baby's breasts and a secretion from the nipples, called witch's milk, is common in both sexes. The infant's breasts should not be massaged, squeezed or treated in any way. The swelling will disappear spontaneously in a few weeks.

5. Breathing—Faint.   All babies' respirations are very shallow and slightly irregular at times. Their breathing is not audible to the average parent. There is no reason to be concerned.

6. Cold and Mottled Extremities.   The extremities will often appear mottled with a faint pink or purple capillary outline. This is due to instability of the blood vessels and is transient in nature. The circulation to the hands and feet is poor. They will feel cold. This is perfectly normal and nothing to be alarmed about. A long night gown and booties are not necessary.

7. Ears.   The ears are composed of soft cartilage at birth. They may be easily bent if the baby sleeps in a certain position. Pinning the ears back is of no value. Once the cartilage becomes firmer the problem will solve itself.

8. Eyes.   There is often hemorrhage into the white of the eye, which is caused by rupture of the capillaries during birth. This blood is absorbed by the body within a week or two. One eyelid may droop or be a little lower than the other. This is called ptosis.

It usually is due to swelling around the eye that impairs nerve function. Ptosis will usually clear spontaneously in a few weeks. If it persists, various surgical procedures are available for its correction.

Pink eye (conjunctivitis) is very common since the infant recently passed through mother's birth canal, which like all parts of the body harbors many bacteria. Routinely, silver nitrate drops or some kind of antibiotic preparation is placed in the baby's eyes as a preventative measure. Most physicians feel silver nitrate has proved to be somewhat irritating and therefore prefer an antibiotic eye preparation.

9. Face—Asymmetry.   Asymmetry of the face, a lop-sided appearance is caused by the position of the baby inside the mother's uterus. The face will become symmetrical by itself in a short period of time.

10. Fever-Dehydration.   Dehydration fever may occur on the second, third or fourth day of life, if the baby's fluid intake has not been adequate. The fever is mild, perhaps only 100 or 100.5 degrees. Upon the administration of extra fluid the fever rapidly subsides.

11. Forcep Marks.   The routine use of forceps to aid delivery has become a standard procedure throughout the United States. Healthier babies are brought forth this way. Sometimes forceps will leave temporary marks on the sides of the face. These areas are red or purplish in color and represent areas of skin injured by forcep application. These marks do not mean that your obstetrician has been rough or less than cautious in any way. They will heal rapidly.

12. Gums—Cyst.   Cysts are pearly white and located on the sharp edge of the gums. They are perfectly normal and will disappear spontaneously without treatment.

13. Hair.   Some newborns are born with thick long wavy hair. The hair is beautiful, but unfortunately most infants will lose most of it. The color of the hair is also apt to change as the baby grows up.

14. Head.   The soft spot on top of the baby's head is called the *anterior fontanel*. This is where the pieces of bone making up the skull will grow together. The size varies at birth from a very small opening to one that may be an inch or more in diameter. The anterior fontanel usually closes between a year and a year and a half of age; occasionally as early as nine months of age. The skin over the fontanel will not break. Do not be afraid to scrub the scalp hard enough to prevent cradle cap.

Most babies' heads are peculiarly shaped after delivery. I mean peculiarly shaped to the parents because they are not round. Actually, what has happened is the head is molded (shaped) from passing through mother's bony birth canal. It will assume a symmetrical shape in a short period of time. No X rays are indicated. No treatment is necessary. No brain damage occurred.

The presenting part of the baby's head, i.e., that part which was delivered first, may become markedly swollen and this is called caput. This spontaneously subsides within one or two days.

The head may also be peculiarly shaped due to a cephalohematoma. A cephalohematoma represents a collection of blood between the bone and its overlying covering called the periostium. Cephalohematomas are caused by pressure of the head against the bony prominences of the mother's pelvis during labor and delivery. Cephalohematomas may be present at birth, but often they are not seen until the second day. Cephalohematomas often feel hard at their margins. This frequently gives the parents the impression that a hole is present in the bone with a mass protruding from it. No treatment is necessary; the lump will go away gradually within six weeks.

15. Neck.   Hemorrhage into the muscles of the neck occasionally occurs in a difficult labor and delivery. The head is pulled down towards the same side as the hemorrhage. If the parents feel carefully enough, they may be able to feel a knot in the muscle. No treatment is necessary as the blood will be gradually absorbed. Sometimes gentle manipulation to stretch the muscle on the affected side will be helpful. Ask the baby's physician to show you how to do this.

16. Pimples.   What appear to be pimples on the baby's face are not. These white pin point raised areas, particularly on the nose, are caused by retention of secretions in occluded sebaceous glands. This normal condition disappears by itself within the first few weeks of life. It is called milia.

17. Scrotum.   In males the scrotum is frequently swollen due to the pressure phenomenon of birth. This swelling gradually diminishes within the first few weeks of life.

18. Skin.   The skin at birth is coated with a thick waxy-like substance. This is very noticeable to the parents if they first see their baby in the delivery room. This waxy-like substance is washed off in the nursery and underneath is the normal reddened skin of the newborn.

19. Startle (Moro) Reflex. A loud noise, or suddenly startling the baby, will cause his arms and legs to raise up and shake. This is called the moro reflex. It is present during the first six months of life because the baby's nervous system is not yet completely developed. The nervous system lacks what is called a myelin sheath. When this sheath develops, at approximately six months of age, the moro reflex will disappear. In some babies this reflex is more noticeable than in others. The shaking that occurs does not hurt the baby. The baby's jaw may frequently shake for the same reason.

20. Sneezing. Babies will sneeze as a means of clearing their upper airway and it does not necessarily mean that they have a cold.

21. Stool. The first stools after birth are composed of material called meconium, which is greenish-black in color. It consists of the waste products which were in the gastrointestinal tract prior to birth. Meconium does not resemble a normal stool.

Occasionally in the newborn period, the muscle around the rectum (sphincter) is very tight. This makes it difficult for the infant to initiate a bowel movement. If this happens the rectal sphincter needs to be stretched by your physician. This is accomplished by a rectal examination on two or three separate occasions.

22. Sucking. Sucking is a normal reflex at birth and continues for some time. Sucking is an instinct. Everything automatically goes into the mouth. The infant even attempts to place his toes in his mouth. This is how the baby learns. Sucking between feedings does not necessarily mean that a baby is hungry.

23. Vagina. In females there is often a slight increase in the size of the genitalia, i.e., vagina. Menstruation which is the result of exposure to the mother's female hormone, estrogen, may occur. This should not be interpreted as bleeding from the rectum. No treatment is necessary.

24. Weight Loss. Newborn babies normally lose between ten and fifteen per cent of their birth weight. Newborns are slow, pokey eaters, and cannot take enough calories to support weight gain until they are a few days old. Some babies will regain their birth weight in three or four days; others will not regain their birth weight until a month of age. A breast fed baby will usually lose a little more weight than a bottle fed baby because the mother's milk supply does not usually come in until the fourth or fifth day.

25. Yellowness (Jaundice).　　Many newborns become yellow after the first twenty-four hours of life. This is called physiologic (normal) jaundice. Babies are born with an excess amount of hemoglobin (blood). The destruction of the excess hemoglobin causes the jaundice. This however, gradually disappears by two weeks of age. It is not harmful to the baby. No treatment is necessary. Jaundice is seen in approximately fifty per cent of all newborns. *Normal (physiologic) jaundice, however, does not occur within the first twenty-four hours of life.* If jaundice occurs before twenty-four hours of age, illness must be looked for.

NOSEBLEEDS

Nosebleeds are a common occurrence when a child has a cold, picks at his nose, or sneezes a lot, with or without nasal allergy. They occur when the mucous membrane protecting the blood vessels that come together at the tip of the nose dry and erode.

Most nose bleeds stop spontaneously. However, ice wrapped in a face cloth applied between the nose and the upper lip is helpful. If the nosebleed continues beyond ten minutes, call your doctor. It may be necessary for him to pack the nose with gauze soaked in adrenalin to constrict the blood vessels. Occasionally, a gauze pack in the back of the nose and throat is necessary. The amount of blood lost always seems greater than it actually is. Do you recall how a drop of ink is absorbed on a blotter? The same principle applies to blood. Acute anemia from loss of blood is a rarity. If bleeding is excessive, your physician will consider various underlying bleeding disorders, such as hemophilia.

NOSE DROPS

Nose drops may be of value anytime there is nasal stuffiness. They play a very important part in the treatment of otitis media. (See Ear Infections.) Many nose drops are available in the drugstore without a prescription, for example, ¼ *per cent Neosynephrine.* In infants and young children, one drop may be placed in

223

each nostril four times a day. In older children, two or three drops may be placed in each nostril four times a day. Saline nose drops, which may be made by adding a pinch of salt to a glass of water, also work quite well in the young child. CAUTION: If nose drops are used excessively, there is a rebound effect. The mucous membranes of the nose become more swollen than before the use of nose drops, thus accentuating the problem. By excessive I mean more than four times a day or for longer than a week at a time. Under these circumstances your doctor should be consulted to treat the underlying problem. (See Colds, Asthma and the Allergic Patient.)

Nose drops must be properly administered to be effective. Lay the child on his back with his head hanging over the side of the bed before inserting the drops. Keep him this way if at all possible for a minute so that the medication can reach far enough back to do some good. A nasal aspirator sometimes works wonders in sucking out the excessive mucous even after nose drops are used. It is a rubber squeeze ball with a glass tip that is inserted into the nose. As the ball expands the mucous is sucked out.

O

OBESITY

Fuel is required by our bodies to meet the demands for work and play. We obtain our fuel from food. The units of fuel in food are called calories. If we eat less fuel than we require we lose weight. If we eat more fuel than we require we gain weight. Our body stores the extra fuel as fat. Our weight is affected not only by how much we eat but also by what type of food we eat. For example, fatty foods contain approximately twice the number of calories as non-fatty foods. A pound of our body's fat is equivalent to 3500 calories: therefore, if we want to lose three pounds a week, we must eat 10,500 calories less. We can burn up some additional calories by planned physical activity, but this is infinitesimal if we are overeating. It has been estimated we must walk thirty-six miles to lose one pound.

A rough estimate to determine how many calories you use a day, is to multiply your present weight by 15, or by 20 to 25 if you are extremely active. Some people eat a great deal and still remain thin; others eat very little and become obese. Everyone is an individual and what we eat must be related to our own body. Pinch the skin on your abdomen or upper arm between your thumb and forefinger. If this measures more than a half inch you are probably overweight.

Most cases of obesity are due to overeating and not to glandular conditions. Those children who have an imbalance in their endocrine glands usually do not have the fat distributed symmetrically over their entire bodies. An important point to remember is that when a boy is obese his penis seems smaller as compared to the rest of his body than it really is. If there is any indication of an endocrine disorder, appropriate tests will be ordered by the child's physician.

Why do children overeat? The reason may be for comfort, pleasure, or love, which was closely associated with food in your child's mind as a baby. Eating food brings happiness to many children so they get in the habit of eating between meals or when they are bored or worried. Sometimes the tendency towards obesity runs in the family.

It is important to watch your weight because there is a definite relationship between health and obesity. Our normal life span decreases markedly when we are overweight. Some hints that will help in reducing weight are to eat slowly, serve smaller portions, avoid fried foods, and weigh yourself weekly on the same scale, at the same time of day, in the same clothing, keeping a graphic record. Parents who merely place their child on a reducing diet may as well give him a joke book. The child must be involved in planning his diet, as well as his parents and physician.

It is important to avoid crash diets because everyone needs a well balanced diet. The fanatical whims of teenagers and fad diets are not based on sound nutrition. If your teenager wants to lose more than a few pounds his physician should be consulted as medical guidance is necessary. For the teenager who wants to lose only a couple of pounds I would suggest any of the many well balanced diets that are available in the grocery store. One of these products may be more pleasing in taste and agreeable to the stomach than another. They provide all the carbohydrates, fats, proteins, vitamins and minerals that are necessary. No nutritional deficiencies will occur. An example is Metrecal, which is sold in cookie, dinner or liquid form. One can of Metrecal four times a day will provide a 900 calorie diet. This allows the child to have three meals and a snack. No other food is necessary. On a 900 calorie diet the average teenager may expect to lose three or four pounds a week.

If obesity is due to a psychological problem and the parents force the child to lose weight, he will quickly regain it. I know of one child who went to a health spa to please her parents and lost twenty pounds. However, she regained it in one month. The desire to lose weight must come from within and not from without. If the gratification obtained by fulfilling oral needs is forcefully taken away the child may develop a tic or behavior problem to replace it.

Objective psychological testing will give the physician some clues about the obese child's personality. Some minor suggestions may create a wholesome environmental background that will lead to more normal eating habits. Psychological testing of one child showed that the mother fed the child as a reward for good behavior. This was solved by involving the child in tasks where he could get approval and gratification from other sources. These tasks may involve the church, scouting, athletics, etc.

There is an example of a 1000-calorie diet under Diabetes. I have suggested this diet to many non-diabetic obese children with excellent results. Pay particular attention to the foods to avoid and list number one which gives foods allowed as desired. The caloric content is divided approximately equally between breakfast, lunch and dinner. I think this is important. The exchange lists certainly make it easy to count calories.

Incidentally, I have carefully studied high protein diets, low carbohydrate diets, weight-watchers, etc. The basic principle is the intake of less calories. If the support of a group is helpful by all means go to weight-watchers, incidentally their cook book is excellent.

When starting a diet, don't expect to lose weight immediately. The body's excess water must be excreted by the kidneys. Most physicians do not believe that pills serve a useful purpose in decreasing the appetite or in getting rid of excess body water. Pills that contain thyroid and digitalis are certainly not indicated.

Once obesity occurs in a child, it is a problem that will require

226

attention the rest of his life. Permitting a child to become fat is a cruelty that sentences him to lifelong isolation and probably will give him a shorter life expectancy.

OBJECTS, FOREIGN—IN THE EARS, NOSE, RECTUM AND VAGINA

Children will commonly insert a foreign object such as a pea, a bead, or piece of paper into openings of their bodies. Parents should not try to remove these foreign objects. Without expert handling they frequently become imbedded deeper in the opening.

Your physician can usually remove such an object by placing a small probe behind it and pulling it out. Small children who do not cooperate may have to be put to sleep in the hospital. The sign of an undiagnosed foreign body in the nose is a one-sided nasal discharge that becomes infected. Children, while exploring, think nothing of placing foreign objects in their rectum or vagina. If the child tells someone he has done this, believe him and take him to the doctor. Scolding and fussing will only draw attention to the matter and make it worse. Treat the problem in a nonchalant manner. Remember the child was not trying to be dirty or act out sexually.

OBJECTS, FOREIGN—SWALLOWING

Children notoriously swallow pennies, nickels, open or closed safety pins, straight pins, and other foreign objects. These objects are usually swallowed without difficulty and pass directly into the stomach. If no difficulty occurred while swallowing the object, your physician will probably not have to see your child. Most foreign bodies move slowly through the gastrointestinal tract without difficulty to be passed out in the stool. It is not necessary for the parents to search diligently in the stools for the foreign body because many times, no matter how careful they are, it will be missed. Rupture of the intestines is almost unheard of. Even chips of glass do not cut the intestines. However, if the patient develops vomiting or abdominal cramps, he should be examined by a physician. Giving a cathartic is of no value. *If choking occurred while swallowing the object, its presence in the airway or lungs must be considered.* An X ray will demonstrate the position of most foreign objects, depending upon their composition. If a foreign object is lodged in the lungs it must be removed. This is done by means of a tube-like instrument called a bronchoscope, usually while the patient is asleep. It is not a dangerous procedure.

OSTEOMYELITIS

Osteomyelitis is an infection of the bone which was associated with a high death rate before modern antibiotic therapy. Although this is no longer true it still presents problems of diagnosis and management.

A. Signs and Symptoms.   The onset is usually sudden with the child appearing quite ill. The fever is usually high. The most important clue is an area of painful swelling localized over a bone. Pressure over the involved area increases the pain. Although any bone may be involved, the commonest sites are the arms and legs. Often there is a history of local injury.

B. Etiology (Cause).   A wide variety of organisms may be involved. However, the bacteria staphylococcus is responsible for the majority of cases. Osteomyelitis usually results from an infection elsewhere in the body, such as impetigo, boils or other infections that were not treated. The infection spreads via the bloodstream to the bone.

C. Treatment.   General supportive measures including strict bed rest, adequate hydration and nutrition, aspirin to relieve pain and control fever, the application of hot packs and elevation of the involved extremity are indicated. Specific therapy is based on knowledge of the causative organism and its sensitivity to antibiotics. X rays are of little value as an aid to diagnosis early in the course of this illness, but are of value approximately three weeks after onset of the disease to demonstrate changes in the involved bone. In all suspected cases multiple blood cultures are obtained in an effort to isolate the organism. However, treatment with penicillin or a combination of drugs is started before the results of cultures are known. Often six weeks of antibiotic therapy are necessary. Occasionally, surgical drainage is required. A favorable response is indicated by the subsiding of tenderness over the involved area.

D. Incubation Period.   The incubation period depends on the child's ability to fight and localize infection. Therefore, it can not be categorically stated.

E. Period of Communicability.   Osteomyelitis is not spread from person to person, but develops as a complication of a wound or infection elsewhere in the body.

F. School Attendance.   When the patient is fully recovered.

G. Prevention.   Obtaining adequate treatment from your physician for all illnesses, but particularly wounds and infections of the skin.

H. Complications.   The infection may become chronic, causing constant destruction of bone with drainage of pus to the outside skin.

P

PACIFIER

I believe pacifiers are a practical necessity at times, particularly for the colicky or thumb sucking baby. It is best, however, not to use the pacifier routinely when the baby is sleeping. Sometimes a baby can become so dependent on a pacifier that he is unable to sleep without it. If the baby is asleep and the pacifier falls out of his mouth, he will probably wake up and scream until it is placed in his mouth again. There are certainly no harmful psychological effects from the use of a pacifier.

A pacifier need not be sterilized. There are millions of bacteria on the baby's skin. When he sucks his thumb those bacteria automatically go into his mouth and he still remains well. A pacifier need only be washed with soap and hot water and rinsed thoroughly before use, even if it falls on the floor.

The decision about the use of a pacifier is made by the parents. They should not be concerned about their neighbor's opinion.

PECTUS EXCAVATUM (FUNNEL CHEST)

Pectus excavatum is a congenital deformity of the chest wall. A depression occurs in the middle of the chest. Some depressions are small, others are disfiguring. The condition often becomes less noticeable as the child grows older. Surgery may be indicated for cosmetic, structural or functional reasons. Ask your physician.

PENIS

A. Emissions—Nocturnal. When the testes have accumulated a quantity of semen, a spontaneous discharge sometimes occurs when the body is relaxed during sleep. The sperm are released in a white sticky fluid. Sexual thoughts or dreams may take place at the time of discharge. This is a normal process and is called either a nocturnal emission (a discharge of fluid during the night) or in slanguage, a wet dream.

B. Erections—Newborn. It is perfectly normal for a new-born baby to have an erected penis. How often have you changed a boy's diapers and noticed this? An erection may occur when the baby's bladder is full or during his bath. There is nothing dirty or sexual about this since adult concepts of sex do not apply.

C. Erections—Spontaneous. Under the influence of certain emotional states the penis may increase in length. Almost every teenage boy has at sometime suffered the unexpected embarrass-ment of having this happen in public. It may be when he is under great stress or tension, when he sees a picture or reads material that is sexually stimulating, when he is dancing with a girl, or even when he is merely standing up in mixed company. Gradually, as he becomes better able to control his thoughts and emotions he outgrows this embarassment.

D. Masturbation (Handling of Penis). The young baby naturally discovers his genitalia just as he discovers his fingers and toes. It is perfectly normal for him to play with his penis for a short period of time. This is how the baby gets acquainted with himself. When a baby discovers his ear lobe he constantly pulls on it too.

Between the ages of three and six, interest in sex is not dormant, contrary to popular belief. Children are naturally interested in each other's bodies. At this age they discover the difference between boys and girls. It is not unusual for children to undress each other or engage in some sort of harmless sex play. They will also hug and fondle their mother and father. Masturbation is not uncommon

230

One of the frequent causes is the fear of something happening to their genitalia. Children do not take for granted the differences between little boys and girls. A girl may imagine that her penis was cut off as punishment, or that it may grow when she is older. A boy discovering that a girl does not have a penis may fear that he himself can lose his penis. Such fears are to be taken seriously. The differences between boys and girls when discovered should not be pooh-poohed. State, "Boys have a penis and when they grow up they will be fathers. Girls have a vagina and when they grow up they will be mothers." Then make a positive statement indicating that you, the parent, are proud that your child has noticed the difference between boys and girls. This will prevent possible confusion in sexual identification. Children should be given an honest answer to all questions so that they do not draw the wrong conclusions from misinformation. To a child any question regarding sex is of no more importance than any question regarding an automobile.

Masturbation is not harmful and cannot cause mental deficiencies or any other defects known to medical science. It cannot cause a child to become psychotic. Do not tell the child to stop masturbating; this only creates guilt and more fear.

Between the ages of six and puberty, there seems to be a dormant period as far as sexual activity or interest is concerned. The child's conscience has become stronger and masturbation is uncommon or infrequent. If masturbation is excessive, it may be due to nervousness and consultation with a physician interested in handling feelings should be obtained. At puberty, or adolescence, masturbation once again increases. Think of the great physical and psychological changes that are occurring at this age. A prominent psychiatrist made the following statement about masturbation— "There are those that do and then there are the liars." Incidentally, masturbation is not confined to boys.

PHENYLKETONURIA

Phenylketonuria is a disease condition that is characterized by mental deficiency and abnormal metabolism of phenylalanine, an amino acid. Amino acids are the building blocks from which protein is constructed.

Phenylketonuria occurs more often in blonde, blue-eyed boys

who have eczema than in the rest of the population. There may be an associated prolapse of the rectum. This is the appearance of the rectal mucosa through the anus. In many states the law requires the physician to perform a screening test on the newborn baby's blood or urine to rule out this condition early enough in life to help prevent mental deficiency. This screening test should definitely be done on your baby. The test is done prior to the baby's discharge from the hospital. It is a simple test to do and does not hurt the baby. During the first week or so of life, the screening test in some cases may be negative even if the baby is affected with this disease. Therefore, it is advisable to have this test repeated in your physician's office at the first monthly checkup. Once the diagnosis is established a special formula is prescribed that is low in phenylalanine, called Lofenalac. Lofenalac is supplied as a powder only. Standard dilution consists of one measure inside the can to each 2 ounces of water. To simplify the job one level 8-ounce measuring cup of powder may be added to a quart of water. This formula will prevent or minimize brain damage in most cases. As the baby grows older certain other foods are added to the diet. These include apples, bananas, blueberries, cabbage, cantaloupe, carrots, celery, cherries, cranberries, cucumbers, grapefruit, onion, oranges, peaches, pineapple, plums, radishes, raspberries, squash, strawberries, tangerines, tomatoes, turnips and watermelon. A special table of permissible foods is available from Mead-Johnson and Company, Evansville, Indiana. At present it is believed that the special diet should be continued until the child is four to five years of age, after which the restrictions may be gradually eliminated.

PILONIDAL CYST & PILONIDAL SINUS

A cyst is a sac containing fluid-like material. A sinus is a narrow elongated recess or cavity. Pilonidal cysts and sinuses occur in the region of the lower back. They appear as a dimple. Clinical signs and symptoms are not present, unless infection occurs. The signs of infection are heat, tenderness, swelling, and pain. This is a rare complication in children, but if it occurs surgical removal of the cyst or sinus is indicated. The best surgical approach is complete excision of the cyst or sinus, allowing scar tissue to fill in the defect.

232

PIMPLES—ACNE

From a medical standpoint, acne seems to be an almost inescapable part of growing up. It is commonest around the age of puberty as the pores of the skin enlarge and more oil is produced. Dirt gets into the larger pores forming blackheads and then secondary infection occurs. Acne is not a sign of impure blood or dirtiness. It has nothing to do with masturbation. Acne is a difficult problem to treat medically. It must be worked on vigorously and with diligence. If acne is not controlled as well as possible, scarring of the face may occur. Plastic surgery may be necessary to correct deep scars. Therefore, it is wise to consult your doctor in most cases.

The single most important principle in the care of acne is not to squeeze the pimples, since this causes the infection to be spread to a larger area and the problem becomes worse. Specific methods of therapy include the following:

1. The use of special soaps such as Fostex and Phisohex. Fostex is available as a soap or cream. Fostex cream is stronger than the soap. Phisohex is available as a soap or cream. Phisohex cream is helpful in drying the oiliness and unlocking the clogged pores. This cream is skin colored so that it hides the blemishes while they dry and heal. The directions for using these medications are printed on the package. These medications are available without a doctor's prescription. They can be used by both boys and girls. Although skin cleanliness is important, the patient should avoid scrubbing the skin raw with these medications. Too much scrubbing only irritates the skin, leaving perforated areas that invite further infection.

2. The avoidance of certain foods such as chocolate and candy is worth a trial period. Almost all skin specialists agree that chocolate should be forbidden food. Foods most often suspected of contributing to acne are nuts, including peanut butter, sweets, fried foods, fatty foods like pork and bacon, spicy foods, carbonated beverages, shell fish and iodized salt. An elimination diet should be tried. Eliminate one or two foods for two weeks and see if the acne improves. Then start eating the food again and see if there is any change in the condition. *Vitamin A—DRY-A*
3. Ultraviolet light. *50000 I. units day.*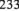

4. The use of antibiotics in special skin preparations, and orally.

5. The avoidance of oily cosmetics, heavy make-up, cold creams or oily hair dressings and ordinary soap.

6. Topical application of Vitamin A acid. WARNING: During the first six weeks of therapy the natural acne process is accelerated, causing a worsening of the clinical picture. After this phase, however, the clinical picture may improve rapidly.

Fortunately as the child develops into adulthood, acne becomes less of a problem.

PINWORMS

Pinworm infestation occurs when pinworm eggs are swallowed with food or drink. These tiny eggs may have been carried through the air to the food, or the food may have been contaminated by unclean fingers. The eggs develop to mature worms in the intestines. Mature female worms then migrate down the large intestine to reach the exterior where they lay their eggs.

The commonest symptom of pinworms is *compulsive itching* about the anus. In children this irritation may lead to nervousness, irritability and lack of sleep. Anemia, picking the nose, or abdominal pain are not signs of pinworms, although anemia and abdominal pain may occur in severe infestations with other types of worms.

Pinworms are white and the size of the head of a pin. They often come out at night. If the parents take a flashlight and spread the child's buttocks apart, they probably will be able to see the pinworms themselves. This is not some horrible disease due to dirtiness. If pinworms are discovered at night or on the weekend, wait until your physician's office hours to call for treatment. The diagnosis may be confirmed by seeing the pinworms under the microscope. A clear plastic paddle that has an adhesive substance on it has been made for this purpose. At night the sticky surface is pressed on the child's skin near the rectum, removed and placed under the microscope the next day. However, many physicians start treatment without laboratory confirmation because this disease is so prevalent in children.

Povan is the treatment of choice. One teaspoon is given for each twenty-two pounds of body weight. Povan is a byproduct of film processing. It is red in color and will stain the clothing permanently.

At times the stool may be stained red. Do not confuse this with blood in the stool. Povan is best given on a full stomach as abdominal cramping and nausea is not unusual. Other medication is available, but is not as effective and requires treatment for a much longer period of time.

A suggested program for the control of pinworms is:

1. Treatment of all members of a household is a practical procedure in controlling re-infection. It has been observed that infection of one member of the family is often accompanied by or followed by infection of several other members of the family, including children and adults.

2. Daily bathing of the anal and adjacent areas with soap and water should be practiced.

3. Frequent washing and scrubbing of the hands, especially before meals, is indicated. Keep the nails short and clean.

4. Avoid putting fingers in the mouth or nose.

Pinworms are often a recurrent problem. The only way to get rid of them permanently would be to treat everyone in the community at the same time.

PNEUMONIA

The air we breath in is carried into the chest by a large tube called the trachea. This large tube divides into a somewhat smaller right and left main bronchus, which go to the respective sides of the body. The main bronchi then divide into still smaller bronchi, at the end of which are sac-like structures called alveoli where the actual air exchange takes place. This is where our blood gives up carbon dioxide and gets oxygen. An infection in the alveoli is called pneumonia. *Bronchopneumonia* or *bronchial pneumonia* are terms that indicate many of the alveoli throughout different parts of the lung are infected. *Lobar pneumonia* is a term that indicates the alveoli in one particular part of the lung are infected. Lobar pneumonia is not as common as it used to be. This probably reflects the control of infectious diseases by antibiotic drugs. Pneumonia, however, is still one of the most common diseases of childhood. Your physician sees many cases a week, particularly in the winter.

A. Signs and Symptoms. Pneumonia may be preceded by a

cold, or develop suddenly, without warning. A cough that becomes progressively worse is usually present. If the parents place their hands on the child's chest they may be able to feel the mucous. Fever is not always present, although a rapid rise in temperature is not unusual. The fever may be continuous or fluctuate. Vomiting may occur. If air hunger develops the child will breathe faster. This is a sign of respiratory distress. Other signs and symptoms of respiratory distress are sucking in of the neck, between the ribs, under the rib cage, and moving in and out of the nose as the child breathes. If not enough air is being exchanged by the lungs, the child will become very pale and eventually blue around the lips. The child may become restless struggling for air.

On physical examination the physician will usually hear rales with his stethoscope. A rale is an abnormal crackling caused by congestion in the lungs. The child's air exchange may be decreased. When the physician hammers on the chest with his finger, dullness may occur. Early in the course of pneumonia the affected areas of the lung may be small and undetectable on physical examination. Thus, an X ray of the chest is indicated when the physician is suspicious of pneumonia, in spite of no objective findings. As a matter of fact, taking an X ray in all proven or suspected cases is extremely good medicine. Interstitial pneumonia which involves the connective tissue holding the lungs together can only be diagnosed by X ray. The white blood cell count may be elevated in bacterial pneumonia. If your child has an elevated white count do not become alarmed. This means he is fighting infection. The white blood cell count is usually normal in viral pneumonia. Blood cultures and cultures of the sputum are obtained in some cases. Cultures may identify the invading organism and help your physician decide upon the treatment of choice.

B. Etiology (Cause). Pneumonia is usually a bacterial or viral infection. The bacteria pneumococcus and staphylococcus are common offenders.

C. Treatment. Most cases of pneumonia can be treated satisfactorily at home unless the child is extremely young or having respiratory distress, as described above. I believe a child under two years of age with pneunonia should be hospitalized because of the high incidence of complications. The drug of choice is based upon the causative organism. This is largely determined by your physician's clinical judgment. Penicillin is usually chosen in pneumococcal infection. Multiple antibiotic therapy is probably indicated against the staphylococcus as it is resistant to many antibiotics. Antibiotics are of no value in viral pneumonia.

The most frequently forgotten ingredient is adequate rest. Children sick with pneumonia must stay quiet watching T.V. or be in bed. Drugs such as aspirin with tempra or tylenol are given to control fever and pain. Cough syrups are prescribed to help relieve this irritating symptom. Nose drops help relieve nasal stuffiness. Milk is avoided since it makes mucous. Liquids are encouraged.

Intermittent Positive Pressure Therapy (IPPB) (inhalation therapy) is a very valuable adjunct to the treatment of acute attacks. I like to describe this as a mechanical cleaning out of the mucous plugs in the lung. With this technique, a machine is triggered each time the patient inhales. This causes air or oxygen under increased pressure, along with any medication that may be prescribed in mist form to be delivered directly to the lungs. The amount of the pressure is adjusted by the therapist. IPPB therapy allows for improved air exchange, more uniform aeration of the lungs and increased bronchial drainage. Treatments may be given as often as necessary.

If your child is hospitalized because of respiratory distress, he will be placed in a tent with cool moisture and oxygen. His breathing will be carefully observed at frequent intervals.

The combination of antibiotics when indicated and good nursing, in addition to the general supportive measures discussed above, almost always lead to a complete recovery. Many children are completely well within seven to ten days. Occasionally two or three weeks are necessary for complete recuperation. Those children who are treated at home without respiratory distress, which is by and large the majority of cases, may only need to be seen in the physician's office two or three times to insure adequate convalescence. Naturally, after recovery common sense measures should be used. The child should not be permitted to go outside and run and play hard every day, but should gradually return to full activity. He should be kept away from people who have colds or other infections until he has a chance to build up his resistance again.

D. Complications. Pneumonia usually heals without leaving scar tissue in the lungs. When a child has completely recovered no

237

physician would be able to tell that he had ever been sick, even if he repeated the chest X ray. The staphylococcus frequently produces thick pus-like material that leads to multiple abscesses throughout the lungs. Rupture of the lung may even occur. Air is then found in the lung cavity. This is called a pneumothorax, which is a true medical emergency. The lung must be re-expanded by placing a rubber or plastic tube between the ribs where it is held in place by stitches and adhesive. The other end of the tube is attached to a suction machine, which gently and slowly sucks the air out of the thoracic (lung) cavity, drains the pus, and allows for re-expansion of the lung. Any child with staphylococcal pneumonia requires hospitalization and needs to be followed by serial X-ray examinations of the chest.

POISONING

With poisoning or accidental ingestion of a foreign substance, take the following steps immediately:

1. Determine what substance was swallowed if possible, and keep the original container.
2. Call your physician, the local poison control center or the hospital emergency room for specific advice as to first aid.
3. Administer first aid according to the advice given.

If advice is not available and no immediate help is available, try to induce vomiting. WARNING: *Vomiting should not be induced if the child is in coma, unconscious, having convulsions or if strychnine, corrosive substances, or petroleum products were swallowed.* Vomiting may be induced by giving a teaspoonful of ipecac every five or ten minutes for two or three doses. The child may also be made to vomit by drinking soapy or very salty water.

The Subcommittee on Accidental Poisoning of the American Academy of Pediatrics recommends that syrup of ipecac and powdered activated charcoal should be available to all parents of young children for possible emergency use in case of accidental poisoning. The administration of these products, however, should be only on the instructions of a physician. An Ipechar Poison Control Kit is available in most drugstores with a prescription. Your doctor will be happy to cooperate. The brown bottle in this kit contains 30 cc's of syrup of ipecac and the black bottle contains 30 cc's of activated charcoal. Ipecac produces vomiting and activated charcoal is a potent absorbent which rapidly inactivates many poisons if it is given before much absorption has taken place. It is effective for virtually all chemicals except cyanide, whether they are organic or inorganic. The activated charcoal is used after vomiting has occurred. The entire bottle of the activated charcoal should be administered to the child followed by large amounts of water or milk. Do not administer syrup of ipecac and charcoal simultaneously because charcoal will inactivate the ipecac.

If your child is in acute distress, he should be brought to your physician's office or the hospital emergency room immediately. Acute distress includes struggling for air, blueness of the lips, unresponsiveness to the spoken voice, convulsions, coma, and shock. Be sure to bring the container from which the child took the poison with you so that the doctor may ascertain for himself how much is left. One important principle to remember is that some of the toxic signs of poisoning may not appear until a few hours later. Do not assume that the product your child has taken is nontoxic if signs and symptoms do not appear immediately. Always consult your physician or the local poison control center if in doubt as to the toxicity of any substance. Your druggist also will be able to tell you about the content of many specific medications.

These common household substances are poisonous: fuel oils, fertilizers, detergents, furniture polishes and waxes, cosmetics, bleaches, alcohol, ammonia, kerosene and gasoline, weed killer, turpentine, pesticides, lighter fluid, lye, medicines including aspirin, paint thinners, and paint removers. Roach tablets are frequently picked up from the floor by children. The commonest one seems to be the Harris Roach tablet, which contains boric acid, which is nontoxic. Thus, the baby or child cannot be hurt by eating any quantity of these tablets. No treatment is necessary. However, many other roach and bug tablets are extremely poisonous.

POLIOMYELITIS (INFANTILE PARALYSIS)

Poliomyelitis is a disease that causes inflammation of the nerve cells, mainly of the spinal cord. Think clearly if there is an epidemic in your community. It is sensible to keep your child away from crowds such as the movies or the local swimming hole, and yet it seems unreasonable to prevent him from playing with his friends. Normal activities should be carried on as far as possible. Schools need not be closed nor their opening delayed. Travel to or from epidemic areas is best avoided.

A. Signs and Symptoms. Poliomyelitis begins like other infections with a sick feeling, fever and headache, followed by a stiff neck. Muscle spasms occur later. *Less than half the cases of poliomyelitis develop paralysis.* Thus, many cases are not even diagnosed, especially when the symptoms are mild like those of a cold and the paralytic aspects of the disease do not develop.

B. Etiology (Cause). Poliomyelitis is caused by a virus.

C. Treatment. No specific treatment is available. Generally supportive measures are used. If respirations become impaired, the patient is placed in a respirator which is a mechanical aid to breathing. If paralysis occurs, physical therapy is helpful in preventing deformities and contractures.

D. Incubation. The incubation period is seven to twenty-one days; more commonly twelve days.

E. Period of Communicability. The period of communicability starts prior to the onset of the first signs and symptoms and lasts through the first week of acute illness.

F. School Attendance. Isolation of contacts is not necessary. The child may return to school with the approval of his physician.

G. Prevention. (See Immunizations.)

H. Complications. If the infection is severe, motor paralysis occurs, followed by a decrease in normal muscle mass of those muscles affected and often by permanent deformities. Respiratory failure may require the use of an iron lung.

PREMATURITY

By definition, a premature baby weighs less than five and one-half pounds regardless of its length of gestation (seven, eight, nine or ten months). Approximately six per cent of all newborns are premature. The causes of prematurity are not known in most cases. Some factors contributing to prematurity are:

1. Advanced age of the mother.
2. Frequent pregnancies.
3. Twins.

240

4. Toxemia of pregnancy. This is a serious illness that occasionally occurs in the pregnant mother, characterized by excessive weight gain, high blood pressure and abnormal urinary findings.

5. Hemorrhage from mother's uterus prior to delivery.

6. Premature rupture of mother's membranes.

7. Accidents.

8. Chronic disease such as tuberculosis, heart disease, or diabetes in the mother.

9. Acute infections in the mother.

10. Congenital malformations of the fetus.

11. Hereditary factors.

The best treatment of prematurity is prevention when possible by adequate prenatal care and general improvement in mother's health through good obstetrical care. The most significant problems that occur in premature babies are:

1. The establishment and maintenance of adequate respirations.

2. The inability to fight infection adequately.

3. Maintenance of a stable body temperature.

4. The inability to digest, hold and absorb adequate amounts of formula.

5. Impairment of renal function.

6. Injury to the central nervous system.

7. Anemia.

The survival rate of premature infants is directly related to their weight. Babies that weigh between fourteen ounces to two pounds three ounces are not expected to live. Occasionally, however, a baby of this weight will survive. Physicians say, "some prematures have it and others do not." The biggest problem at this weight is that the body organ systems are not capable of adjusting to their environment. Those that do survive probably have body systems which are better developed than others of the same weight. Babies weighing between two pounds three ounces to three pounds five ounces have a fifty per cent chance of survival. Babies weighing between three pounds five ounces to four pounds six ounces have a seventy-five per cent chance of survival. The survival rate for babies between four pounds six ounces to five and one-half pounds is not significantly different from full term babies. The chief causes of death in the premature infant are:

1. Congenital abnormalities.
2. Hemorrhage into the brain.
3. Infection.
4. The respiratory distress syndrome (RSD). (See separate heading.)

The first twenty-four hours of a premature baby's life is the most critical period of time because this is when most of those babies who will not survive pass away. The next most critical period of time is the second twenty-four hours of life. After the first forty-eight hours of life death is infrequent.

A special problem may occur in very small premature infants called retrolental fibroplasia. Retrolental fibroplasia causes blindness and is due to excessive oxygen concentration in the incubator. Occasionally this problem is unavoidable if the infant is to survive.

The four cardinal principles in caring for a premature infant are:

1. Provide adequate oxygen.
2. Maintain a stable body temperature.
3. Prevent infection.
4. Provide adequate nutrition.

The comprehensive care which your premature infant receives includes the following: At delivery, appraisal and resuscitation, placement in a heated nursery unit, care of the cord and eyes, and proper identification. A physical examination within the environmental controls of the incubator with positioning, stimulation of respiration when necessary, oxygen when necessary, maintenance of warmth, protection from infection, nothing to eat orally for twenty-four to seventy-two hours, followed by a special formula every two or three hours, with special attention to nutrition thereafter. During hospitalization repeated physical examinations, comprehensive nursing care and continued care in the incubator are given. Graduation to a regular crib, preparation of the parents, and discharge home with medical follow-up follows. Most physicians believe that a premie is ready for discharge when he weighs between five and five and a half pounds and he is on a four-hour feeding schedule. Mother should get used to her baby by feeding him before discharge. Parents also need to discuss their feelings about prematurity with their physician. There probably was a great let-down when their baby was left in the hospital. Because of the special care the baby has been given, the parents may lack self-confidence, feeling the infant is extremely fragile. This is not so. By the time a premie is ready to go home he need not be treated any differently than a full term infant.

The growth and development of a premature baby will be slower than that of a full term baby, and the more premature the baby is, the slower the expected growth and development. This is perfectly normal. It has been medically proven that many years are actually necessary for the premature baby to catch up with the full term baby. From the standpoint of body chemistries and physiology, this may not occur until the teens. Your baby, however, has not lost any capacity to grow and develop because he was premature. Mentally and emotionally he is normal.

PSYCHIATRY AND PSYCHOLOGY, CLINICAL

A psychiatrist has received a medical degree and then specialized in dealing with emotional problems. A child psychiatrist is specifically trained to deal with children.

Clinical psychology deals with the science of behavior. Clinical psychologists have received a master's degree or a doctor's degree in their specialities, which includes psychotherapy, diagnostic testing, and research. A psychologist differs from a psychiatrist in that he cannot prescribe drugs. Most clinical psychologists insist that their patients have a complete physical check-up by their medical doctor before treatment is started. This helps prevent the psychologist from treating a child with an emotional problem due to some underlying physical condition. Most psychiatrists also follow this procedure even though they are capable of giving a physical examination themselves.

Both psychiatrists and psychologists use special techniques to deal with children, such as play-therapy. Dolls are used to represent different members of the family, and they speak for them. Soon the child becomes involved and speaks for the dolls too.

A person's physical health affects his emotions and vice versa. The human body must be treated as a whole. The mind cannot be divorced from the rest of the body. For example: If a person becomes extremely angry, adrenalin is released into the blood stream that prepares his body for flight or fight. Here emotions affect physiological functions. If a person has asthma, he may become concerned about his death as he struggles for air, which may make his asthma worse. In this example, something of a physical nature helped shape attitudes and feelings.

There is no stigma attached to visiting a psychiatrist or psychologist and discussing your problems with them. Going to these doctors does not mean that you are crazy. A crazy person is one who is psychotic and not oriented as to time, place, and person. All normal people have certain minor problems in different areas; if these minor problems begin to become acute, a psychiatrist or psychologist can help if you are willing to help yourself. It is extremely difficult to solve many of these problems by yourself, because of your own defenses. The problem may be denied or projected to someone else. Support is also needed as the problem is resolved. Look upon these specialties as preventive medicine. Human beings have the tendency to make the same mistake over and over again when it comes to emotions and feelings. The only way to prevent this is to be able to look at yourself objectively. This can only be accomplished with a trained doctor who is able to prevent his own feelings from coloring interpretations. Such a person is a psychiatrist or a clinical psychologist trained in psychoanalysis.

Surveys indicate that seven per cent of pre-schoolers are in need of some psychiatric care. The importance of this statement is overwhelming, since by the age of six most major mental mechanisms have been formed. Thus, children's mental health is largely dependent upon the early years. When indicated, parents can provide no greater service to their children than proper referral to a psychiatrist or psychologist. Whether the child's behavior problems are the result of brain damage, or of neurotic attempts at adjustment, their correction at an early age can prevent further maladjustments that could extend into adult life. It is an investment for the future. Children who do not receive the necessary treatment will become obviously ill, later.

When consulting these specialists, parents certainly are entitled to ask what progress is being made from time to time. However, the therapist cannot tell you exactly what the child says; that is privileged information. This is necessary for the continuance of a good doctor-patient relationship. How long will therapy take? It is almost impossible to give an estimate, but the sooner the problem is dealt with, the quicker the resolution.

If the services of a psychiatrist or psychologist cannot be honestly afforded, social agencies may provide family counseling or child guidance which is invaluable. Unfortunately, the demand for services is far greater than trained personnel available, which usually causes many time delays.

PSYCHOLOGICAL TESTING—HOW TO PREPARE YOUR CHILD

Now that you have decided (or perhaps been persuaded) that your child needs a psychological evaluation in order to determine if he has some psychological problem, how do you explain this to him? A visit to the physician or dentist is not too difficut to explain on the basis of need, but you do not want your child to think you believe there's something wrong with his "head." In spite of a great deal of continuing education in the field, there are some individuals who feel there is a stigma attached to going to a psychologist.

There are many factors to be considered here. One of the most important is your own attitude. If you are fearful or apprehensive, the child can sense this. There may also be some feelings of guilt— "What have I done wrong?" Most parents do make mistakes, but these are, for the most part, honest mistakes. Very few parents deliberately hurt their children. Something has gone wrong and you want to know what. This is a healthy step in the right direction and should help some of the guilt feelings you may have.

There is no need for apprehension. Psychologists are not "witch doctors" nor mind readers. They are individuals trained to use tests and interviews to try to get at the causes of the problems and not to sit in moral judgment. Their aim is diagnosis and recommendations for the type of help their test results indicate is needed. This can range from psychotherapy to remedial academic help. As a rule, the psychologist will want an interview with the parents first to get a developmental history and to obtain an idea from the parents as to what they think the problem may be. If possible, both father and mother should be present.

Since rapport is important for valid test results, it is important that the child have some idea as to whom he is going to see. He

245

should not go in expecting to have his teeth filled or to get a shot of some type.

The age of the child will affect the type of explanation you give him. So will the nature of his problem. For a young child, under six or seven, it is probably better to tell him he is going to see a nice person who will play some games with him and talk to him. This is true; tests for younger children are so designed as to seem like games.

The older child, from around seven to twelve, should be told he is going to have some simple tests, but that they are different from school tests since there is no reading or writing. Unless the child is quite severely mentally retarded he is probably aware that he is having some problems, either at school or at home. He may very well be unable to admit that he has any problems, but try to explain to him that you would like to find out if he has and if there is anything you can do to help him. The idea of the psychologist being a person helpful to both you and him should be stressed. Once again, your attitude here is most important. Try to relieve both his and your anxiety as much as possible by being as matter of fact about the appointment as you would about a visit to the dentist or physician. Try to avoid the implication that he is "crazy" or that there is something vitally wrong with him.

Adolescents are probably the most difficult group to whom to explain the need for psychological testing because they are most prone to feel it is the family who is out of step and not they. They are also old enough to feel that having to go to a psychologist is embarrassing. With this age you have to be firm and insistent. Although the adolescent will probably deny the existence of any problems, point out the reality of the school or home situation to him, again avoiding the implication of it being anyone's fault. Even if a teenager threatens to tell the examiner he is "dumb" and not to take the tests, parents must get him to the psychologist's office. The doctor is trained to handle this type of situation. If the teenager absolutely refuses to go to the psychologist's office then there is the problem of who is in control.

Try not to make too big a thing out of the visit to the psychologist at any age. Don't tell the child days in advance as he would have a chance to sit and worry about it. This too depends on the age of the child. Older children need a day or so advance notice, but this is not essential for the younger child. If the child appears to be somewhat embarrassed and shy about going, it is not necessary to tell the other children. Children can be cruel.

Remember that you are not alone in having a child who seems to be having psychological problems. It is estimated from reliable research that from five to fifteen per cent of all children need psychological help at some time during their development years. The sooner a problem is diagnosed and remediation begun, the more chance there is of clearing up the problem. If minor difficulties can be caught early, they can often be prevented from becoming major problems later in life. The tendencies toward delinquency and to drop-out can start with frustrations in school or at home at a very early age.

Try to remember also that there can be some problems occurring over which you really had little or no control and, yet, which you now have to cope with and help your child cope with. As a trained expert, this is the psychologist's job and he will help you if you will permit him to do so.

Tests

Psychological tests are divided into two main types, individual and group. These types in turn have two main divisions, intelligence testing and personality evaluation. Group testing is exactly what the name implies. These tests are given to all children at school to determine their academic achievement in order to see if they are learning as they should. These are usually administered once a year. Group intelligence tests are generally given every two years. These tests are helpful in giving some indication of the child's mental ability. They are not as exact a measure as individual tests. Many school systems also give tests for school readiness. It is very important that the child be ready for school mentally, emotionally and physically so that he will not be confronted with tasks that are beyond him, and get off to a poor start. A chronological age of six does not necessarily mean that the child is automatically ready for first grade. Individual psychological testing should be done by a trained psychologist. Indications for having this done are suspected differences from the normal, either much lower or much higher, lack of academic achievement although intelligence appears normal,

247

signs of emotional problems, physical symptoms with no medically ascertainable causes, inability to get along with others, etc. There are very few areas which do not have psychologists in private practice to whom you can take your child if you are concerned about his problems. Be sure to check out training and qualifications. Most states now have certification for psychologists. In addition, most modern school systems have psychological services to which the principal or teacher can refer you.

Types of Individual Intelligence Tests

These tests are administered on a one to one basis with just the psychologist and the child present. It is better if the parent is not present since this can be distracting and perhaps affect the test results.

1. Stanford Binet. This test compares chronological age with mental age in order to figure out the I.Q. (intelligence quotient). The mental age is divided by the chronological age usually expressed as a multiple of 100. The intelligent quotient of a ten year old whose mental age equals that of the average 12 year old is 120. The Stanford Binet is usually used with younger children below the age of seven if they have intelligence within the normal range. It is used as an alternate test for other individual intelligence tests or with older children who are suspected of being mentally handicapped. There is no reading or writing on this test. Items start with simple tasks which the normal two year old can perform and gradually become more difficult. The child continues until he fails six items in succession. Some of the items require ability to talk and others depend upon manual ability and visual-motor coordination for success. This was one of the earliest individual tests designed to measure intelligence and is still widely used.

2. Wechsler Intelligence Scale for Children (WISC). This test is divided into two halves, verbal and performance. The first half measures the ability of the child to show his fund of knowledge and to express his thought processes verbally. There is no reading or writing. The examiner presents the question orally and records the answers in writing. This is valuable with children who are intelligent, but who, because of their inability to read, do poorly on the group intelligence tests at school. The performance half of the WISC requires little or no verbalization, but consists mainly of visual and/or manual problems which also require intelligence to solve. This is helpful in determining the intelligence of children who have difficulty in expressing themselves verbally. The two scores are combined and prorated to determine the I.Q.

3. Wechsler Adult Intelligence Scales (WAIS). This is used for adolescents and adults and is given at age sixteen and up. The format is essentially the same as the WISC.

4. Wechsler Pre-School and Primary Scales of Intelligence (W.P.P.S.I.). This is a fairly new intelligence test similar to the WISC, but with simpler items and is designed to be used with children who are not old enough to handle the items on the WISC. It is a downward extension of the WISC and as such is valuable for follow-through if testing needs to be done again when the child is older. There are a few other intelligence tests, but they are not as widely used nor as well proven. There are differences of opinion as to whether parents should be told the exact I.Q. Inasmuch as the I.Q. is merely a number, it is generally considered more beneficial to explain the test in detail, pointing out the child's assets and liabilities. Test results should always be interpreted to parents and recommendations should be made based upon the test findings.

Individual Personality Testing. Probably one of the most widely used tests is Projective Drawing of the Human Figure. Just as a novelist puts something of himself into his writings, the child puts something of himself into his drawing of people. This test is useful in discerning the child's attitude toward himself and his perception of his own body image. Careful screening by a trained individual can reveal a great deal of helpful information. It can also be useful as a tool for a rough approximation of intelligence. Family drawings are also used. The child is asked to draw a picture of himself and his family. From this his perception of his place in the family constellation and his interaction with the other members can be hypothesized. For example, a younger sibling may loom up as the largest figure in the family. This is, of course, not the reality of the situation, but it is the child's perception of it and therefore reality for him. In this way a clue can be obtained as to what may be one cause of his difficulties.

The Bender Motor Gestalt Test. This is another widely used individual test. Easily administered, it consists of a series of nine geometric designs which the child is asked to copy. This test when used in conjunction with some of the subtests on the WISC is helpful in picking up clues to difficulties in visual motor abilities; not so much visual acuity as trouble with reversals, directionality, etc. It is also useful in giving clues to neurological problems.

The Children's Apperception Test (C.A.T.). This consists of ten pictures of animals in various family situations. The child is requested to tell a story about each picture and from this story clues are picked up (much as in the Family Drawing) which help the psychologist to ascertain if there are problems within the family which may be partially responsible for the child's difficulties. This test is used mainly with children under ten years of age.

The Thematic Apperception Test (T.A.T.). This is similar to the C.A.T. mentioned above except that the pictures are of people in many different situations. It is more likely to be used with older children, adolescents, and adults. The child is requested to make up a story about each picture. There are twenty cards, but as a rule only ten to twelve are presented, depending on the nature of the problem. The rationale is the same as with the C.A.T. It is given in order to find out the causes for the problems and to find out how the child is attempting to cope with them.

The Rorschach Psychodiagnostic Test. This is probably the best known of the individual personality tests, due to widespread publicity on T.V., magazine articles, etc. It consists of ten cards, each with a relatively different constructed ink blot. The child is asked to tell the psychologist what the card looks like to him or of what it could remind him. The cards are presented twice. The second time the child is asked to explain, if he can, why he sees the card as he does. This is a very helpful tool in getting at some of the personality dynamics and in obtaining an idea of how the child perceives and reacts to his environment. As a word of caution, however, more training and practice are needed for the proper administration and interpretation of the Rorschach than the other tests previously mentioned.

In all individual testing the psychologist records the responses in writing and as a rule makes behavioral notes as to the child's reactions to him and the testing situation. Of course, all these tests are not administered to each child. It is up to the discretion of the psychologist to determine which tests will best aid him to diagnose the problem.

In summary, if your doctor or you as a parent feel psychological testing is necessary, be sure you find a qualified individual to do the testing and the interpretation. The tests are good, but only as good as the person using them. The main purpose is to diagnose the problem and find the causes. Before any recommendations can be made this must be done. There is no point in going for psychological help if you are not planning to follow through on the recommendations. This would be as foolish as going to your lawyer and then ignoring his advice. If the psychologist finds a problem, be prepared to go along with his recommendations for remedying it.

PURPURA—IDIOPATHIC THROMBOCYTOPENIC (BLEEDING INTO SKIN)

This disease is characterized by bleeding into the skin. The small pinpoint hemorrhages are called petechiae and the larger areas of hermorrhage, ecchymoses. Idiopathic thrombocytopenic purpura is due to a deficiency in blood platelets, which are necessary for normal clotting. The exact cause of the platelet deficiency is not known. Idiopathic thrombocytopenic purpura may follow the administration of antibiotic, if an unexpected reaction on the patient's part should occur. The diagnosis is proven by examination of the bone marrow where the platelets are formed. This disease usually responds rapidly to treatment with steroids (cortisone). If necessary, a platelet transfusion may be given to stop the bleeding. If your physician is suspicious about a particular drug causing this illness, he will avoid that drug in the future. Occasionally the disease can recur, but this is unusual. The outlook for complete recovery in seven to ten days is excellent.

R

RABIES

Rabies is an infectious disease of animals usually transmitted to man by the bite of a mad or rabid dog. Few physicians have had experience with this disease as it is extremely rare, and preventable.

A. Signs and Symptoms. There is always the history of an animal bite. This bite is followed one week to several months later by numbness and tingling of the involved area that lasts for one or two days. This is followed by either irritability and excitation or depression. Muscle spasm, particularly of the throat, occurs at the mere sight of food or water. Thus, the term, hydrophobia. There is increased salivation. The temperature is elevated. Finally convulsions, paralysis, coma and death occur.

B. Etiology (Cause). Rabies is caused by a virus and transmitted by the bite of an animal that is infected or rabid. This is not necessarily a dog. Rabies has been isolated in wild foxes, bats, rats, etc.

C. Treatment. The only treatment is prevention by proper care and control of dogs and other domestic animals. The rabies vaccine is of no value once the disease has developed. Approximately twenty per cent of persons who are bitten by animals known to be rabid have developed rabies if not treated with the rabies vaccine. However, rabies rarely occurs unless the individual actually has been bitten by the animal. If an animal bites your child, report it to the local health department and consult your physician. If the bite occurs when the health department is closed, it should be reported to the police department. Your local health department has adequate personnel and proper procedures for finding the offending animal and observing it for the necessary period of time. The animal bite is treated like any other cut. (See Cuts.)

The World Health Organization Expert Committee on Rabies has considered various types of exposure to rabies and made the following recommendations:

1. If contact with the rabid animal has been indirect, or if there has been only a lick on abraded skin, no exposure is considered to have occurred and vaccine is not recommended.

2. If the exposure was mild, i.e., a lick on abraded skin, or on muscosal surfaces, or for single bites not on the head, neck, face or arm:

    (a) If the animal was healthy at the time of exposure, withhold vaccine, but observe the animal for ten days.

    (b) If during the ten-day observation period the animal is proved to have rabies or becomes clinically suspicious, start vaccine immediately.

    (c) If the animal has signs suspicious of rabies at the time

252

of exposure, start vaccine immediately, but stop injections if the animal is normal on the fifth day after exposure.

(d) If the animal is rabid, if it escapes or is killed, or if it is unknown, give complete course of vaccine. If the biting animal is wild, also give rabies antiserum.

3. If exposure was severe (multiple or single bites on the head, neck, face or arm) the indications for giving vaccine are the same as in mild exposure. (See 2 above.) In addition, in every category, the administration of rabies antiserum is recommended.

Although the most recent report of the World Health Organization Expert Committee on Rabies recommends the use of rabies antiserum, there is evidence that serum administered concurrently with vaccine seriously interferes with the development of active immunity. If serum is used, the Committee recommends supplementary doses of vaccine ten and twenty days after the last usual dose.

The minimal course of treatment consists of one subcutaneous dose daily for fourteen days. It is recommended that the injections be made under the skin of the abdomen (belly) on alternate sides each day. Each dose should be given in a site not previously used for the vaccine.

Another variation in dosage should be considered for persons bitten by wild animals. Such bites are followed more frequently by the development of rabies than are the bites of domestic animals; furthermore, in these circumstances, the disease is likely to have a shorter incubation period. To provide protection as quickly as possible, the early administration of additional amounts of vaccine is advisable. Therefore, after the bite of a wild animal, whether or not antiserum is given, it is suggested that two doses of vaccine be administered daily for seven days, followed by one dose daily for another seven days. This makes a total of twenty-one doses of vaccine. The supplemental doses recommended by the World Health Organization at ten and twenty days after completion of the initial series are also indicated, particularly if antiserum has been used.

A duck embryo (dried killed rabies virus) vaccine has also been manufactured. Experiments have shown that duck-embryo tissue contains little or none of the "paralytic factor," and thus the incidence of neurological side effects has been low.

Inasmuch as the early development of protection is important and the risk of neurological reaction after the administration of duck-embryo vaccine is minimal, a useful modification of the usual dosage schedule consists of starting duck-embryo vaccine immediately in any patient bitten on the head, neck, face, or upper extremity by a suspect animal. If, subsequently, on the fifth day the animal is healthy, the vaccine may be discontinued pending further observation.

D. Incubation Period. The incubation period is usually one to three months.

E. Period of Communicability. The disease may only be spread by the bite of an infected animal and not from man to man.

F. Prevention. (See Treatment.)

G. Complications. The disease is fatal.

RASHES

The purpose of this section is to give parents some clues as to the cause of various rashes. *Refer to the specific disease entity for confirmation, except as stated below:*

1. Chicken pox. The rash starts as a clear blister on a red base. The blister becomes filled with pus. A scab is formed which falls off and leaves a scar. Lesions are found in various stages at the same time.

2. Cold Sores, Fever Blisters, Herpes Simplex. The gums are red and sometimes bleed. Small blisters develop which quickly rupture, leaving ulcerated areas which become covered by grayish-white plaques.

3. Coxsackie Virus. This virus, in addition to being the cause of some common colds, may cause a flat to slightly raised rash very similar to measles.

4. Diaper Rash. This is a flat red rash that is usually confined to the diaper area. It may appear over night or in a matter of hours. Secondary invasion by a fungus is common, giving the edges a scalloped appearance.

5. ECHO Virus. This virus, in addition to being the cause of some common colds, may cause lesions similar to chicken pox, except that they are much smaller in size and usually fewer in number.

6. Eczema. The acute form is characterized by redness, itching and oozing. The chronic form is characterized by a dry, scaly skin with a tendency to crust formation. Scratching may produce bleeding and secondary infection. It is most common on the face, behind the knees and in front of the elbows. Eczema usually occurs before the age of six.

7. Erythrema Multiforme. Large red welts of various sizes and shapes appear. The rash frequently comes and goes.

8. German Measles. The eruption appears on the face first, spreading rapidly over the entire body in a few hours, after the onset of swollen glands in the neck. The rash is flat, pink, and tends to remain discrete. It resembles measles the first day, scarlet fever the second day, and fades on the third day.

9. Hives. Hives are characterized by large welts that suddenly appear. They may vary in size and shape over a number of hours.

10. Impetigo. Impetigo is characterized by raised blisters on a red base. The blisters become filled with pus which later forms thick yellowish crusts. The rash spreads by autoinoculation, secondary to itching.

11. Measles. The rash of measles appears on the face and works its way downward towards the feet. It is a flat, red rash that itches. Fever is always present when the rash breaks out and persists. The eyes are red and coughing commonly occurs.

12. Molluscum Contagiosum. Small elevated, waxy pearl-like lesions are present, without other signs of illness. This is a self-limited disease that requires no treatment. However, removal of the molluscum bodies by squeezing them will promote rapid healing. There is no discussion of this condition elsewhere.

13. Prickly Heat. Prickly heat is seen mostly in warm weather when there is excessive perspiration. It is a fine raised rash that usually occurs over the shoulders and neck and in the folds of the skin. No associated signs of illness are present.

14. Poison Ivy. A history of contact with the plant may be obtained. The plant is distinctive since there are three leaves on a common stem. The rash is characterized by small, clear, red blisters that itch intensely. (See Contact Dermatitis.)

15. Rheumatic Fever. A flat, red rash that may vary in size, and shape found on the belly wall sometimes occurs. There are always other associated signs and symptoms such as fever, arthritis, and the history of a sore throat that was not treated.

16. Rheumatoid Arthritis. A flat, red rash may suddenly appear with the occurrence of fever and rapidly subside as the fever disappears. The individual lesions are transitory even if the rash persists. Typically, there are red swollen joints—most often the knees, fingers and feet. (See Arthritis.)

17. Ringworm. Ringworm is characterized by well demarcated circular lesions. If the scalp is involved, the hairs in the area lack luster or are very brittle. The hairs are often broken off close to the scalp so that the affected area appears bald.

18. Rocky Mountain Spotted Fever. There may be a history of a tick bite. Three days after the onset of illness a rash appears which starts on the extremities and spreads over the rest of the body. The rash is red and raised with a tendency to become hemorrhagic.

19. Roseola. High fever (104-105 degrees) occurs for a few days. In spite of this, the child does not act sick. He frequently continues to play. When the fever breaks a rash appears on the chest and stomach before quickly spreading to the rest of the body. If the parents are not specifically looking for the rash, it may be entirely missed as it may disappear in a matter of hours.

20. Scabies. Scabies is characterized by burrowing under the skin and associated severe itching.

21. Scarlet Fever. The rash of scarlet fever is like a red flush. Pallor around the lips is prominent. Increased red lines appear in the elbow region. The tongue has a typical strawberry appearance. The rash may feel sandpapery like the rash of prickly heat. The patient in most cases appears acutely ill, with high fever and a sore throat.

22. Smallpox. All the lesions of smallpox are in the same stage at the same time. This is contrary to chicken pox in which the lesions are present in various stages at the same time. No additional knowledge is necessary to recognize this disease. Therefore, it is not discussed elsewhere except under immunizations. Most physicians have never seen a case.

23. Tinea Versicolor. This is a superficial fungus infection of the skin. Areas of depigmentation are present that look like "white spots." The involved areas rapidly spread. Specific treatment is available by prescription. There is no discussion of this condition elsewhere.

24. Typhoid. Rose spots may appear at the end of the first week. This red, flat to raised rash appears in crops, usually over the abdomen (belly) and back. Fluctuating fever is usually present.

RESPIRATORY DISTRESS SYNDROME (RDS)

The failure of the newborn infant to make the necessary transition to adequate respirations after birth is called the respiratory distress syndrome, regardless of its cause. There are many theories as to the mechanisms that initiate the newborn's respirations, but none have been actually proven. Spontaneous respirations may be delayed for a number of seconds and this is of no clinical significance. However, respirations delayed beyond two minutes at birth indicate a serious problem. The normal respiratory rate in the newborn is approximately forty breaths per minute, and the respirations are often slightly irregular.

The respiratory distress syndrome is characterized by rapid breathing. There may be sucking in in the neck, between the ribs, under the rib cage and moving in and out of the nose as the infant breathes. The baby may look blue. Respiratory distress may be present at birth or may not become apparent for a few hours or a few days. The incidence of respiratory distress is higher in premature infants, in infants where there have been prenatal maternal complications, such as diabetes, in women who have had repeated pregnancies, and in babies born by Caesarean section.

The principal causes of the respiratory distress syndrome are:

1. Prematurity.
2. Pneumonia.
3. Hyaline membrane disease.
4. Damage to the central nervous system—brain hemorrhage.
5. Atelectasis

The respiratory distress syndrome is responsible for, or contributes to, approximately 50 per cent of all infant mortality.

The best treatment is prevention. Adequate prenatal care is the best prophylactic means and prevention of a difficult labor and

257

delivery where possible by proper obstetrical management. (See separate headings.) The rarer causes of the respiratory distress syndrome are discussed below:

1. Atelectasis. Contrary to popular belief, the lungs do not completely expand with the first cry. They expand gradually over a period of approximately a week. Atelectasis means that some parts of the lungs are not expanded for adequate air exchange. If enough of the lung tissue is not expanded, the respiratory rate increases as the baby attempts to get enough oxygen. There is no specific treatment for atelectasis of the newborn. All supportive measures, including the use of oxygen, control of temperature, maintenance of adequate fluids and prevention of secondary infection, are important. The most critical period of time is the first forty-eight hours of life. It is during this time that those babies who do not survive are most apt to pass away. An outlook of guarded optimism is indicated. Each additional hour that the baby breathes enhances his chances of survival. Many physicians have seen children who breathed one hundred times a minute survive.

2. Pneumothorax. Air in the thoracic cage (chest cavity) prevents complete expansion of the lungs, thus causing respiratory distress. Pneumothorax may be caused by underlying disease of the lung, over-enthusiastic resuscitation of the newborn or rupture of a cyst. The diagnosis is confirmed by X ray. Treatment consists of the early aspiration of the air from the chest cavity by means of a needle or a plastic tube to which constant suction is applied. With early recognition and treatment the outlook is favorable.

3. Diaphragmatic Hernia. Diaphragmatic hernia is characterized by absence of some of the diaphram muscle which separates the chest cavity from the abdominal cavity (belly). Part of the baby's intestines extend up into the chest cavity. The severity of the respiratory symptoms depends upon the degree of protrusion of the contents of the abdominal cavity into the chest cavity and the resultant amount of lung tissue collapsed. The belly appears unusually flat. The clinical impression is confirmed by X ray. Surgery is the only possible treatment. The outlook is not favorable.

4. Choanal Atresia. Choanal atresia is a congenital obstruction that occurs between the back of the nose and the throat, which prevents the passage of air through the nose. One or both sides of the nose may be involved. In the presence of symptoms of respiratory distress the diagnosis may be easily ruled out if a small plastic tube will pass through the nose into the back of the throat. If blockage occurs on both sides, immediate surgery is indicated. If the blockage is one sided, surgery is postponed until the infant is gaining weight and doing well. Treatment usually results in a favorable outcome.

5. Aspiration of Meconium or Aminotic Fluid. Aspiration of meconium (stool-like material) from the intestinal tract of the infant, or of aminotic fluid (that which surrounds the baby in utero), usually produces sudden distress. The diagnosis is confirmed by X ray. Since this condition occurs prior to birth, the outlook for the baby depends on the severity and duration of the oxygen lack prior to delivery.

RHEUMATIC FEVER

Rheumatic fever is a disease that involves many different parts of the body. It should not be confused with rheumatism, which is any disorder of the extremities or back characterized by pain and stiffness.

A. Signs and Symptoms. The symptoms may be acute or so mild that there is little indication to consult a physician. The possible symptoms include:

1. A slightly elevated temperature or a high fever, easy fatigability, tonsillitis or sore throat.

2. Arthritis, which involves primarily the larger joints and migrates from one joint to another.

3. Inflammation of the heart, which only your doctor can diagnose by an increased heart rate, development of heart murmurs or an abnormal rhythm. In more serious cases, the heart may become enlarged and heart failure may develop.

4. Purposeless movements known as chorea.

5. A flat, red rash that may vary in size and shape, frequently found on the belly wall.

6. Fibrous nodules most frequently found around the joints.

7. Recurrent nosebleeds.

8. Shifting abdominal pain that eventually confines itself to the upper left side of the abdomen (belly).

After recovery from the acute attack, recurrences are possible if your physician's instructions are not accurately followed. Any of the above signs and symptoms may be present during another attack. If the diagnosis is suspected, most physicians will hospitalize the patient. An adequate workup includes an electrocardiogram, a chest X ray, a sedimentation rate, which is a non-specific blood test to determine if any active disease process is present, a white blood cell count, urinalysis and cultures of the nose and throat.

Certain criteria have been established that must be met to make the diagnosis of rheumatic fever. These guidelines were established because the medical profession does not want to make the diagnosis on a random basis since the implications as to life span, insurability and job procurement may be permanent. Parents should not jump to the conclusion that because their child has a sore throat and arthritis, he has rheumatic fever. Certainly, your physician needs to be consulted.

The incidence of rheumatic fever is higher in a climate characterized by cold, dampness, and sudden variability of temperature. It is also more commonly found in environments of poverty, poor hygiene, and malnutrition. Some families are more susceptible than others. There is a seasonal rise in the incidence of rheumatic fever along the eastern seaboard in the spring and on the west coast in the winter.

B. Etiology (Cause). Rheumatic fever is caused by an allergic reaction to a streptococcal infection.

C. Treatment. All streptococci present must be eradicated. The drug of choice is penicillin. My favorite is long acting bicillin as it lasts the necessary fourteen days which is required to eradicate all streptococci. Other antibiotics are available for those children who are allergic to penicillin. Aspirin has been used for many decades in the treatment of acute rheumatic fever. The response of fever and joint involvement is dramatic. Aspirin may even be used as a therapeutic test to differentiate the fever of rheumatic fever from that caused by other illnesses. Some authorities use aspirin for many weeks, but this probably is not necessary. Toxic side effects may occur from aspirin because of the high dosage required in this illness. The toxic manifestations include:

1. Ringing in the ears.
2. Nausea.

3. Vomiting.
4. Headache.
5. Little areas of bleeding under the skin.

If these effects occur, the drug is temporarily discontinued, and then restarted at a lower dosage schedule. Other drugs are available if the child cannot tolerate aspirin. Steroid (cortisone) is frequently used. There is a wide variation in the duration of therapy and recommended dosage. Most physicians feel that steroid should be reserved for the more serious cases, and not used routinely. There is no specific therapy available if inflammation of the heart occurs. It has been suggested that steroids may terminate the inflammation of the heart, but this has not been proven. Bed rest is most important. It may even have to be prolonged if the heart is severely involved. Most physicians believe that bed rest should continue for a period of approximately two weeks. Following this, the patient may be permitted up and about indoors with at least two rest periods a day, one in the morning and one in the afternoon. At the end of this time the child may gradually increase his physical activity so that he may return to school approximately six weeks after the onset of illness. Patients who have had a recurrence of rheumatic fever require a longer period of bed rest. Often these children must stay out of school for three to four months. The rest required in the early stages precludes the child from doing school work in the hospital. The child must be encouraged to express his feelings about his illness and more particularly about bed confinement. It is very difficult to maintain strict bed rest, particularly when the child is without symptoms. The type of therapy must be individualized for each child. In children with severe involvement of the heart, congestive heart failure may occur. The usual treatment is digitalis and diuretics, which help the kidneys get rid of the excess body fluid that accumulates. If chronic heart disease develops that leads to an irregular rhythm, special medications are available. Surgical treatment may be necessary in rare cases. It is important that a consistent long-term approach be used. The child should see a physician at regular intervals so that all the advances of modern medicine can be used to help him.

D. Incubation.   Rheumatic fever occurs approximately ten

261

days to three weeks after an untreated or inadequately treated strep infection. The child must be seen early when a strep infection occurs if the physician is to prevent complications.

E. Period of Communicability. Rheumatic fever per se is not a communicable disease but only stereptococcal infection is highly contagious until treated.

F. School Attendance. School attendance is not to be permitted until the child is completely well, as determined by his physician.

G. Prevention. This consists of adequate treatment of all streptococcal sore throats. This means that if your child develops fever and a sore throat, he should be examined by a physician during the course of his illness. After an attack of rheumatic fever the patient must take prophylactic penicillin or prophylactic sulfa for the rest of his life. *It has been proven that both of these antibiotics, if given faithfully every day will prevent recurrent streptococcal infections and thus another flareup of rheumatic fever.* Testing urine specimens for penicillin excretion in 136 rheumatic children on penicillin prophylaxis revealed that only 32% showed compliance during all test periods. No one is perfect. Therefore. I recommend that children with rheumatic fever receive a shot once a month of long acting penicillin called "bicillin." Then no slip-ups can occur in the program to prevent recurrent rheumatic fever.

Children with rheumatic fever who must undergo tooth extraction should be protected with additional penicillin.

RICKETS

Rickets is a disease characterized by softening of the bones. Bowed legs are typical. Enlargement of the elbows, knees and ankles may also occur. A protuberant abdomen is not uncommon. Rickets is due to a deficiency of vitamin D. The diagnosis may be established by determination of the blood, calcium and phosphorus level. X-ray examination of the wrists presents a typical appearance in advanced cases.

The treatment consists of an adequate daily intake of vitamin D until the laboratory studies return to normal. Healing usually occurs within two months and is complete with early and sufficient treatment. Mild bone deformities tend to heal spontaneously with age.

262

With the addition of 400 international units of vitamin D to each quart of milk in the United States, and other vitamin fortified foods such as cereals and margarines, vitamin D deficiency is extremely rare as long as some semblance of a reasonable diet is maintained. Although rickets should always be considered in the extremely malnourished child, parents should not blame cases of normal bowing or knock knees on rickets. (See Bowed Legs & Knock Knees.)

RINGWORM

Ringworm is a contagious skin disease which is characterized by well demarcated circular lesions. It most frequently occurs in the scalp, but may be found anywhere on the body. In the scalp the affected area appears bald as the hairs are broken off and lack luster.

Ringworm is a fungus infection. The diagnosis is confirmed by use of a special light, which will identify the affected hairs. Microscopic examination of the hair and skin scrapings or cultures, may also reveal the fungus. Your doctor should be consulted. Ringworm is difficult to cure. Specific ointment is available for treatment. If necessary, a special antibiotic may be taken orally. The period of communicability is unknown. Ringworm is spread by clothing or direct contact. School attendance is permissible as long as the patient is receiving treatment, providing a stocking cap is worn. Prevention consists of personal hygiene.

ROCKY MOUNTAIN SPOTTED FEVER

This disease is named Rocky Mountain Spotted Fever (RMSF) because it was first found in the Rocky Mountain area of the United States, but it is certainly more widely spread than that.

A. Signs and Symptoms.   RMSF begins with chills and fever, headaches and muscle pains. Three days after the onset of illness a rash appears which starts on the extremities and spreads over the rest of the body. The rash is red and raised with a tendency to become hemorrhagic. Fluctuating fever may be present for a number of weeks. A history of a tick bite is significant.

B. Etiology (Cause).   A specific disease organism, which is transmitted by the bite of a tick.

C. Treatment.   Specific antibiotic therapy is available to combat the infection. The outlook for complete recovery is excellent.

D. Incubation Period.   About one week.

E. Period of Communicability.   Since this disease is spread by the bite of a tick, it is not contagious.

F. School Attendance.   When completely recovered, as designated by your physician.

G. Prevention.   (See Immunizations.)

ROSEOLA INFANTUM

Roseola is a very mild contagious disease, usually confined to children less than three years of age.

A. Signs and Symptoms.   The onset of this illness is sudden, with a rise in temperature to 104 or 105 degrees without any apparent cause. The child may be slightly irritable or listless, but does not act as ill as you would expect. The child frequently continues to play. Convulsions are commonly precipitated by the high fever. (See Convulsions.) When the fever drops to normal a rash appears. The rash is red and flat, and appears on the chest and stomach before quickly spreading to the rest of the body. It may disappear in a matter of hours. Unless the rash is specifically looked for it is often missed by the parents.

B. Etiology (Cause).   Roseola is caused by a virus.

C. Treatment—Control of the Fever in Order to Prevent Convulsions.   Aspirin with tempra or tylenol is used to control the fever. (See Aspirin, Tempra, Tylenol.) If necessary cold alcohol baths may also be given. Occasionally an injection of fever medication must be given by your physician to bring the temperature down. This does the job in twenty or thirty minutes. Antibiotic is of no value since this is a viral infection.

D. Incubation.   The incubation period is seven to seventeen days.

E. Period of Communicability.   The period of communicability is probably from twenty-four hours prior to the onset of fever until the temperature returns to normal.

F. School Attendance.   The child may attend school when he has been without fever for forty-eight hours.

264

G. Prevention. None. One attack probably confers permanent immunity.

H. Complications. Seizures, especially in an infant who has had febrile convulsions in the past.

ROUND WORMS

If your child passes a worm in his stool that looks like an earthworm, do not become frightened. It is probably a round worm. The diagnosis is established by seeing the worm or finding eggs in the stool. It is not a serious problem and treatment may be safely delayed until your physician's regular office hours. Specific oral medication is available that is effective and only necessary for two consecutive days.

S

SCABIES

Scabies is a contagious parasitic disease of the skin. It is characterized by severe itching that is often followed by secondary infection. The most common locations are the lower part of the body. It is caused by the itch mite which burrows into the skin. Treatment consists of benzyo benzoate, twenty-five per cent, applied after a bath while the skin is still moist. Once the original application dries, it is repeated. A second bath is taken twenty-four hours later. If itching still persists, treatment can be repeated in one week. Antibiotics are prescribed if secondary infection occurs. All contacts are treated, and infected clothes and bed linens sterilized.

SCARLET FEVER AND STREP THROAT

There is no difference between scarlet fever and a strep throat, except one. The bacteria, streptococcus, produces an exotoxin. If the child is allergic to this exotoxin, he develops a rash and hence the diagnosis of scarlet fever. If the child is not allergic to this exotoxin, no rash occurs and the diagnosis is strep throat. Therefore, there is no medical justification to be more frightened of scarlet fever than a strep throat. The peak incidence occurs among the five to ten year olds; the infection is uncommon in children under three years of age.

A. Signs and Symptoms. Symptoms usually include a sore throat, fever, headache and sometimes vomiting. In many cases the sore throat is the outstanding sign. In most cases the patient appears acutely ill with high fever. Unfortunately, the above signs and symptoms may be absent or equivocal often enough that some cases go undiagnosed. If a rash is to develop, it usually appears twenty-four to forty-eight hours after the throat becomes sore. It is a flat, red rash, somewhat similar to a red flush. The rash may feel like sandpaper. Pallor around the lips is prominent as the rash does not involve this region. Increased red lines may appear in the elbow region. The tongue has a typical strawberry appearance. In a climate with seasonal changes strep infections peak in March or April with the lowest incidence in August.

B. Etiology (Cause). A bacteria known as the streptococcus.

C. Treatment. *Penicillin is the drug of choice and should be given for ten to fourteen days.* The omission of one or two doses may lead to complications which otherwise are preventable. Therefore, I heartily recommend an injection of long acting penicillin (known as bicillin) that will last the necessary length of time. Then there can be no slip-ups. Occasionally, there is soreness around the site of the injection when bicillin is given. Some children may even limp for a day or two. This occurs because bicillin must be given deep into the muscle as it is slowly released and absorbed. If the patient is allergic to penicillin other suitable antibiotics are available. The medications provide one of the few miracle cures in medicine. An acutely ill child will be almost well in forty-eight hours. Complications should not occur if the diagnosis is made and therapy instituted early enough. To the best of my knowledge there has never been a strep infection that has not responded to penicillin.

D. Incubation. The incubation period is two to five days.

E. Period of Communicability. The period of communicability starts with the first signs and symptoms of the illness and lasts until all abnormal discharge from the nose and throat has stopped—until all the streptococci have been eradicated.

F. School Attendance. The child should not attend school until a physician has determined that he is completely well. Con-

266

tacts need not be quarantined. Parents should not become alarmed if they receive a notice that their child was exposed to scarlet fever in school, because the chances of catching it are slight.

G. Prevention. There is no known immunization to scarlet fever. A medical expert on strep infections has recommended that brothers and sisters of the ill child receive preventive doses of penicillin because the exposure is within a small family group. I subscribe to this recommendation. If a child in the family should already have rheumatic fever and be on preventive penicillin, the dosage should be doubled.

H. Complications. Nephritis and rheumatic fever are the major complications. They usually occur two to three weeks after the fever is gone. *These complications are serious, but preventable with early treatment of all strep infections.* To be doubly sure, most physicians recommend that the child's heart and urine be checked two or three weeks after the child is supposedly well. (See Nephritis and Rheumatic Fever.)

SCHIZOPHRENIA

Schizophrenia is a severe mental disturbance. The signs and symptoms are regression in behavior, loss of interest in one's surroundings, bizarre movements, repetition of movements, and disturbance of speech. The child is autistic—everything seeming to come from within himself. The child's ideas bear no relationship to his environment. Schizophrenia is a psychosis and, therefore, the child may not be completely oriented at times as to time, place and person. The exact cause is unknown. However, it is known that schizophrenia is not hereditary and does not result from such things as masturbation or anything the parents may or may not have done during development of the baby in mother's uterus. It may be metabolic in origin. The treatment of choice is psychotherapy. Unfortunately, when problems are this serious the outlook is not hopeful. Confinement to a private or state hospital specializing in mental illness may be necessary.

SCHOOL FAILURE

There are many reasons why children fail in school. The first thing to be considered is whether some physical problem such as hearing loss, defective vision or chronic illness exists. Physical problems are ruled out by a complete physical examination and appropriate diagnostic tests when indicated. Some children fail because they do not have the basic brain power. Their I.Q. should be determined. If emotional problems are suspected, psychological testing is essential. A conference should be set up between the parents and teacher and, if necessary, the principal.

Ideally, every child before attending school, in my opinion, should receive psychological testing and I.Q. determination. Unfortunately schools have arbitrarily stated that children enter first grade at the age of six and certain rules are made that this age must be obtained within so many months of September 1st. Obviously, this is not the best way of determining when your child is ready for school. Private testing with a clinical psychologist before starting school is ideal.

Some children fail in school because they are bored. They are extremely bright and the tasks required may be too easy. They are not challenged by the work. If your child seems unusually bright and this is proven, see that reference material such as the *World Book* or *Junior Encyclopedia Brittanica* is provided at home. Additional work might also be assigned by the teacher to enable the child to obtain a richer background.

If the child is extremely nervous in school, a tranquilizer may help. I do not object to the use of tranquilizers, but one must remember they are treating a symptom and not doing anything about the cause of the tension. If the tension continues or becomes worse, objective psychological testing is mandatory. A problem can be solved in a short period of time if it is attended to early, just like the repairs on your automobile, but if the problem persists for a long period of time, it will become more complicated, more imbedded and more difficult to treat.

Some children may be doing poor work in school because they are over-conscientious. Other children are accused of doing poorly because on the surface they appear lazy. Actually, those things which children like to do they will do well, providing they have not been pushed too hard and the parents are not too critical of their accomplishments.

Many so-called good children are underachievers because they have difficulty in dealing with their own feelings of aggression. They are poorly motivated. The child is often depressed, has difficulty in self-assertion and uses passive resistance to authority.

268

If your child is graded with S's for satisfactory and N's for not satisfactory on his report card in the early years of grade school do not become upset if he gets an N or two occasionally. Acknowledge the "S" and "N" without being critical. He knows what they mean. Certainly his report card should not be compared with that of another child. If a child needs to be tutored in a special subject, fine, but try to use a professional tutor. The methods of teaching have changed and the scope of material enlarged. Parents are emotionally involved with their child and are bound to lose their tempers occasionally. This does not help the child.

Learning Disabilities—The Interjacent Child— Minimal Brain Damage

Some children who do poorly in school have no obvious damage to their nervous system. However, very subtle clues may be present that indicate there is minimal brain damage that is causing difficulty with learning. These children do not quite fit into special schools as presently constituted as they have normal intelligence quotients. However, they are incapable of satisfactorily responding to the regular school program. Thus, they live in a shadowland of muddled perception, impoverished language development, and disorganized thought structure. The child may experience distorted sound patterns, but he is not deaf. He may be visually impaired, but he is not blind. Emotional disturbance may have erected a barrier to an effective school experience, or in turn further maladjustment may have been created by the child's failure to perform satisfactorily in the regular school program. The interjacent child is out of step. The public school system may say about this child: "We cannot understand him, he is capable of doing the work but he simply won't." The parents may be frustrated because their child appears bright but they say: "he is too lazy and stubborn when it comes to school work." This type of child can definitely be helped if his learning disabilities are discovered early enough and corrective steps taken.

Although symptoms are present during pre-school years, the typical youngster does not begin to be much of a problem until he begins school when pressures begin to build. The youngster must now perform certain tasks in specified ways at definite times. Why all of a sudden are we discovering these youngsters? Probably because society is demanding more and more of each generation. These children can be taught and will learn. A few public school systems have special programs for them, and there are a number of excellent private schools throughout the country. It was recently estimated that five million children in the United States fall into the interjacent category. (See Dyslexia.)

SCHOOL PHOBIAS

The child is afraid to go to school. He prefers to stay home because he believes that while he is in school his parent or parents will leave him. *This is a psychological emergency.* The child should definitely have definitive treatment from a clinical psychologist or child psychiatrist. Parents must not think that a school phobia is something the child will outgrow. School phobia will only get worse if professional help is not obtained. While this professional help is being obtained, the child must be made to attend school. The child should be reassured, however, that if he wants to come home from school early, the parents will come and get him when he calls.

SINUSITIS

The sinuses are cavities in the bones that drain through small passageways into the nose. They occur on each side and are named as follows: The frontal sinuses just above the eyebrows in the forehead, the maxillary sinuses in each cheek bone, the ethmoid sinuses above the inner passages of the nose, and the sphenoid sinuses behind the nasal passages.

Only the maxillary and ethmoid sinuses are well enough developed in children to be of practical consideration. Infection involving the sinuses is called sinusitis. The symptoms may be acute with fever and pain, or there may only be a postnasal drip. Postnasal drip is caused by mucous and pus draining into the nose from the sinuses and dripping down into the back of the throat. Although the cough it creates is annoying, this is far better than the material entering the lungs.

On physical examination there is often acute tenderness to moderate pressure over the sinuses. A light can be shined through the

270

sinuses in a dark room to see if they transluminate. If the light does not shine through the sinuses, one can assume they are filled with fluid or pus.

Sinusitis may be either viral or bacterial in origin. It is usually a complication of an upper respiratory infection, sore throat, or tonsillitis. The organism that caused the primary infection usually causes the secondary infection of the sinuses. Repeated attacks may be due to allergy.

Treatment consists of antibiotics for bacterial infection, antihistamines, nose drops, as well as rest, adequate fluid intake, and medication for fever and pain. Surgical drainage of the sinuses is rarely indicated since the advent of modern antibiotic therapy. Skin testing is necessary for repeated attacks due to allergy. (See Asthma and the Allergic Patient.) Recovery from sinusitis is rapid and complete. It is not a serious problem in children.

SLEEP

Contrary to popular belief, babies do not just sleep and eat, but are awake a good part of the day. But each baby is an individual; many babies require more sleep than others. As long as the baby is healthy and is growing and developing normally he is getting enough sleep. Do not use your own need for sleep as a guide.

The daily amount of sleep needed decreases with advancing age. Infants under fifteen days of age typically sleep for sixteen hours a day. Unfortunately some infants don't know the difference between day and night because it is a learned response. By the twelfth week of life a sleeping pattern is usually developed with sleep concentrated at night.

A baby should be put to bed at a regular time preferably right after eating. That is when the baby is most contented and willing to sleep. No special precautions such as tiptoeing around the house need to be taken. The baby that is used to a noisy house will not be bothered and the baby that is used to a quiet house will only be bothered if it is especially noisy.

It is better for the baby to sleep on his stomach. That way if he should vomit he will not aspirate food into his lungs which may cause pneumonia. Also the head is relatively heavy and constant pressure on the back of the head from its own weight might make the head fairly flat temporarily. The baby that sleeps on his stomach seems to have a more symmetrical head, as he rests his head on both sides.

Many babies are awakened by bright sunlight. To prevent this, use a shade or some sort of dark blind. After waking up many babies fuss for a few minutes, but if left alone develop the habit of amusing themselves.

A separate room for the baby is preferable from birth on. If this is not possible, he certainly should not sleep in his parent's room after six months of age. It is surprising in psychoanalysis how often children recall intercourse between their parents. The child often believes the mother is being attacked. In addition, the baby that sleeps in his parents' room too long becomes too dependent upon the arrangement and the older he is, the harder it is to break the habit.

A baby may accidently start waking up at night after he has been awakened for medication, or received extra attention while sick. He has become used to it and likes it. The only way to cure this is to let him fuss and cry it out. Babies have to learn there is nothing to be gained from this type of behavior. If the baby cries all night after waking up, as long as you know he is not sick, hungry or hurt, let him cry. He cannot rupture his lungs. If you give in after one hour of crying he will test your will power each night for longer periods of time. Always bet on the baby under these circumstances.

During the first two years of life the infant gradually lengthens his nighttime sleeping habits and his waking daytime periods. By the age of two years a child may sleep an average of twelve hours at a stretch. However, rigid rules regarding a certain number of hours of sleep do not make sense. Many three year olds will not actually fall asleep until eight o'clock at night even if they are put to bed at 7:30. Yet, they will wake up at six A.M. If the child is not fussy the following day and is well behaved, it is obvious that he has gotten the proper amount of sleep. Generally speaking, I find that most children will nap twice a day until two or three years of age. After that time they will not actually go to sleep. The best that can be accomplished then is a quiet peaceful period where they may sit or lie on their bed and look at a book or play with a favorite toy. This is worthwhile because it does provide necessary rest and prepares them for the continuance of their day.

There is nothing wrong with sharing a bedroom with another child of the same sex. Unfortunately, one child may not be able to sleep as long as he would like under these circumstances.

A child should never be allowed to sleep in his parent's bed. It may seem the simplest solution at the time, particularly if the child is anxious and nervous, but it is difficult to get him to give up this security. The child should be brought back to his own bed and reassured. Talk with him and try to figure out what is bothering him.

It is not necessary to keep children's doors open. If they are afraid put a night light in the room. However, do not let the child become overly dependent on it. If this begins to happen, there needs to be communication on the subject between the parents and child. The underlying reason for the need of a night light must be found. A child that becomes afraid of the dark could have this fear persist into adult life.

For the young child fear of separation is great, particularly if the mother is starting to work. This fear is most acute at bedtime. The child may fight going to bed by crying or screaming for hours after being put there. He may only be quiet when mother is sitting next to him. Give him time to become adjusted to this new fear. Begin by going out for an hour, and then returning. This will allow the child to become adjusted to a babysitter. Mother's quick return reassures the child that she will always return. Then the time can gradually be increased.

If parents already have a two year old fearful about going to bed at night, ask your doctor for a sedative. Phenobarbital is commonly used; however, this causes excitation in some children. Therefore, my favorite sedative is chloral hydrate suppositories. A child, by sheer will alone, may counteract any sedative. If this is the case, it may be necessary to sit at the child's side until he is fully asleep.

The best treatment is prevention. When excuses are used to avoid going to bed, such as asking for a drink of water or for permission to go to the bathroom, say "No, you just had a drink of water" or "No, you just went to the bathroom." Tell him where mom and dad will be in the house in case he really does need anything. A two year old child will frequently climb out of bed by

273

himself and go to wherever the rest of the family is. At this time, he will be particularly cute because he realizes that he must perform if he is to stay up with his parents. Many parents may think that the child is being cute and permit his presence. However, once the child is put to bed, the child must be made to stay there. If the child continually gets out of bed, purchase a fish net and cover the crib. This net is put on matter-of-factly. There should be no indication that the child has been bad or is being punished.

SNAKE BITES

Poisonous snakes found in the United States are the rattlers, copperheads, moccasins, and coral. The bite of a venomous snake is really an injection in which hollow fangs deposit venom in the skin. It leaves two small puncture marks and pain occurs at the site of the bite. Take snake bite kits on all camping trips where poisonous snakes are found. Emergency first aid consists of some type of constricting band placed between the wound and the body. Do not apply the tourniquet tightly as its purpose is to slow blood flow, not stop it. At the site of the bite cross cuts are made three-eighths of an inch in depth to induce bleeding. Suction through these cuts is then applied by mouth or suction cup. Specific treatment consists of injection of antivenom by your physician as soon as possible to neutralize the poison.

SORE THROAT (PHARYNGITIS)

Pharyngitis is inflammation of the back of the throat.

A. Signs and Symptoms. The onset is usually acute with fever. The presence of pain in the back of the throat is difficult to determine in young children. Tiredness, abdominal pains and vomiting may also be present. When the child is examined the back of the throat is beefy red and swollen. The tonsils are often involved.

B. Etiology (Cause). A sore throat may be either a viral or bacterial infection.

C. Treatment. I believe any child with a sore throat should be seen by his physician. A streptococcal sore throat may have serious complications if left untreated. The cause cannot be determined over the telephone. (See Scarlet Fever—Strep Throat.) The antibiotic of choice is based upon the causitive organism as determined by your physician's clinical judgment. Antibiotic is of no value in a viral infection. If the child is old enough to gargle, a preparation such as S.T.37, which is available in the drugstore without a prescription, is of value. Mix an equal amount with water and gargle four times a day. If the child is too young to gargle, one squirt of Chloroseptic Spray four times a day may be used. This is available in the drugstore without a prescription. Both these preparations relieve pain. Take tempra or tylenol and aspirin for fever. (See Aspirin, Tempra, Tylenol.) Rest and additional fluids are also important. All the suggestions made under Treatment of the Common Cold may also be helpful at various times.

D. Incubation. The incubation period depends upon the specific organism causing the infection.

E. Period of Communicability. This depends upon the specific organism causing the infection.

F. School Attendance. The child may return to school when he has been without fever for forty-eight hours or permission has been obtained from his physician.

G. Complications. Usually there are no complications, except in an untreated streptococcal infection. (See Scarlet Fever—Streptococcal Sore Throat.)

(SPINE) SPINA BIFIDA, MENINGOCELE, MENINGOMYELOCELE

Spina bifida is a congenital abnormality caused by incomplete fusion of one or more of the vertebra in the back. Occasionally through this defect there will be a protrusion of the meninges which cover the spinal cord. This is called a meningocele. If some of the spinal cord also protrudes through the defect, it is called a meningomyelocele. The protrusion of the meninges and/or spinal cord occurs approximately once in every one thousand births.

Most cases of spina bifida are uncomplicated and not associated with clinical signs or symptoms. The diagnosis of spina bifida may be confirmed by X ray. Occasionally, a special dye is injected into the spinal cord to facilitate X-ray studies.

Cases of spina bifida without symptoms, if diagnosed, need no treatment. The presence of a meningocele or meningomyelocele is obvious at birth. If the nerves of the spinal cord are involved, the bladder and bowels are affected as well as the muscles below the lesion. There would be constant dribbling of urine and stool. Surgical excision and plastic repair are indicated in all cases of a simple meningocele. Surgery is indicated in some cases of meningomyelocele, depending upon the general condition of the baby and whether there are any other congenital abnormalities present. The outlook is guarded as these children already have a neurologic disability of varying severity and nothing can be done to replace the damaged tissues.

SPINAL TAP (LUMBAR PUNCTURE)

Under sterile conditions with local anesthetic a needle is placed between the lower spines in the small of the back. Fluid is then withdrawn from the spinal canal and sent to the laboratory for analysis. This is the same procedure frequently used in obstetrics for anesthesia, except that after the spinal fluid is withdrawn an anesthetic agent is used to replace it.

In children with unexplained fever or signs of meningitis the risk is slight compared with its value in establishing a specific diagnosis.

Side effects include backache, headache, vomiting, and a stiff neck. However, these side effects occur in only five per cent of the patients and are mild and temporary. If your doctor suggests a spinal tap, agree to it.

SPLINTERS

A small splinter near the surface of the skin may be safely removed by the parents. Sterilize a sewing needle by holding it in an open flame. Press the needle against the skin at the point of the splinter. Scrape and dig gently to push the splinter out.

SPRAINS

A sprain is characterized by swelling around the joint and some limitation of motion. Before moving the child, support the joint by placing the extremity on a pillow.

It is impossible for your doctor to have X-ray vision. Almost all sprains should be X-rayed. This is the only sure way to rule out the possibility of a fracture. A fracture need not be a major break, but may simply be a chip or small bend. Nevertheless, these fractures need to be immobilized for an adequate length of time to ensure healing. (See Broken Bones.)

If no fracture is present the sprained part may be supported by an ace bandage. Aspirin is given for pain. The swelling may be brought down faster by elevating the affected part above the level of the heart. This allows the tissue fluid to leave the affected area more rapidly. The skin around the sprain will become black and blue because of the bleeding that has occurred under it. Two to three weeks are required for this discoloration to disappear. Sometimes enzyme pills prescribed by your physician will help promote the re-absorption of this blood. Naturally, the more opportunity the child has to rest, the faster healing will occur. Normal activity such as going to school can be permitted unless the sprain is painful, but athletics should be prohibited. Do not confuse sprained joints with a charley horse. A charley horse is a slang expression for an athletic injury that represents a pulled (strained) muscle.

STEROIDS (CORTISONE)

Steroids are wonderful drugs that may be life saving when properly used. They are widely used in acute rheumatic fever, rheumatoid arthritis, asthma, inflammatory diseases of the eye, nephrosis, hives, eczema, certain blood diseases, and in certain cases where the body does not produce enough cortisone.

There are as many different steroid preparations on the market as antibiotics. The dosage and side effects of each are slightly different. The particular steroid that your physician chooses will depend upon his clinical experience and the advances being made almost daily in steroid therapy.

Steroids should not be used indiscriminately or for prolonged periods of time unless absolutely necessary. There are some undesirable but reversible side effects. If a patient has been receiving steroid regularly it must be slowly withdrawn when indicated, to prevent withdrawal symptoms.

STOMACHACHES—ACUTE & CHRONIC

A. Acute.   With an acute stomachache the possibility of appendicitis always exists. An appointment to see your physician within a reasonable period of time should be obtained. Be sure to bring a urine specimen to your physician's office; he may want to check it. The child may not be able to urinate at the particular time it is necessary to collect the sample.

The commonest cause of abdominal pain in children is an upper respiratory infection (cold) and not appendicitis or food poisoning. *One cardinal rule is never give an enema or anything that will cause vomiting before the child is examined by his doctor.* A careful physical examination will reveal the cause of acute belly pain in most cases. At times a blood test may be indicated. The treatment depends upon the cause. If the stomachache is secondary to infection elsewhere, that infection must be properly treated. If a surgical condition of the abdomen (belly) is present, surgery is indicated. (See Appendicitis.)

B. Chronic. Chronic stomachaches are a frequent problem. Kidney infections, ulcers, intestinal allergy, and psychological problems are common causes. Providing the child's physical examination is normal and the history is not compatible with a specific illness, most physicians will prescribe some type of antispasmodic to relax the intestinal tract. However, if the stomachaches become more severe and frequent, a complete workup, including X rays of the kidneys, stomach, and intestines is in order. It is surprising how often a congenital abnormality of the kidney or an ulcer is found. If the diagnostic workup is normal and the pains continue psychological testing is indicated.

Many parents ask if worms can cause stomachaches. The answer to this is "yes," but it must be a very severe case. I really do not believe that pinworms, which are almost universal, can cause any significant amounts of abdominal pain.

What about the child who complains of stomachaches at feeding time? Is this an excuse not to eat? The pain to this child is certainly real, but one must look at what the pain means. It probably means that the child is tense and nervous. Possibly mealtime is being handled in less than an ideal way. The child-parent relationship must be carefully studied.

STUTTERING

Stuttering is very common and there can be a variety of causes. It may be due to tension or to a new environment. Tongue-tie has nothing to do with stuttering. It is more common in boys, and often runs in families. Some days the stuttering will be worse than others.

278

Most two year olds who start to stutter will outgrow it by themselves in a few months. Do not be concerned about speech training at this age. If the problem persists and becomes progressively worse, a clinical psychologist or child psychiatrist should be consulted.

SUDDEN DEATH (CRIB DEATH)

Newspaper articles frequently report that a baby goes to sleep in good health, but suddenly passes away. For this reason sudden death seems more common than it is.

When an apparently thriving infant is found dead in its bed, the shocked and disbelieving parents almost invariably ask "What did I do wrong?" "Could I have prevented this?" "Did my baby suffocate?" Although medical authorities do not always agree about the causes of sudden death in infants, much is known. Many of these cases are due to interstitial pneumonia. This is a rare type of pneumonia that may be present with very few symptoms; thus the parents and physician do not know the baby is ill.

The old idea that thymus enlargement could cause sudden death is no longer tenable medically.

The idea that the child died of suffocation is the most difficult one for the parents to dispel. Because the child is frequently found with the blanket pulled over its head, it is natural for them to suspect suffocation. This is unlikely, however, as sudden death occurs primarily among male babies between one and four months of age, usually in the winter and spring, and almost always during sleep. It has also been proven that covering the face of infants with ordinary bedding is not sufficient to cause lack of oxygen. Babies are also capable of raising their heads at birth from a prone position, adding further proof to the fact that sudden death is not due to suffocation.

I want to assure parents that there is nothing they can do to prevent this rare but unfortunate happening. If it occurs they must face life again; there is no justified reason to feel guilty. If guilt persists a clinical psychologist or psychiatrist should be consulted.

SWOLLEN GLANDS (ADENITIS)

Since it is difficult to determine the cause of swollen glands, with the exception of mumps, over the telephone, most cases should be seen by your physician. This is particularly so if fever is present or if the child is getting progressively worse. When a child has tonsillitis or pharyngitis there are numerous lymph glands in the neck which may swell in an effort to prevent the spread of disease. A principal sign of German measles is markedly enlarged glands in the back of the neck. Infection of the glands may also occur as a primary disease, i.e., the only disease present. Sometimes abscess formation occurs.

The treatment depends upon the underlying cause. If tonsillitis, pharyngitis, or a primary disease is present, appropriate antibiotic therapy is indicated. No treatment is necessary for swollen glands caused by German measles. The use of an old-fashioned ice collar is of no value. It should be emphasized that once the glands in the neck swell, it may be many weeks or many months before they will completely return to normal size. Often a little scar tissue will remain in the gland. If the parents feel the back of their necks carefully, they will probably be able to feel little lumps, which represent the remnants of swollen glands. This is perfectly normal, and does not represent cancer.

T

TEETHING

The average baby gets his first tooth at approximately six months of age. He is teething most of the time during the first two and a half years of life as twenty baby teeth appear. Some babies may be fretful for three or four months and drool a lot before the first tooth comes in. Other babies will have no problems and all of a sudden one tooth will appear. Sometimes babies will have four or five teeth appear at the same time. Under these circumstances the parents can understand why babies may become extremely irritable at times.

Babies who are teething seem to enjoy having their gums massaged. Massage them between your thumb and forefinger for five minutes every day, or when necessary. Dip your fingers in paregoric if the infant is really fretful. Many parents ask if the gums can be cut to relieve the pain of teething. This is no longer recognized as acceptable medical treatment.

Teething is blamed for entirely too many illnesses in children. I cannot accept a fever above 101 degrees from teething, unless teething has precipitated an infection. Ear infections are frequently associated with teething since an excessive amount of mucous is usually present.

The teeth usually appear in the following order:

(a) Two teeth in the middle of the lower jaw. These are called the lower, central incisors. Incisors are the name given to the eight front teeth which have sharp, cutting edges.

(b) The four upper incisors.

(c) The two remaining lower incisors.

(d) The four first molars. There is a space left between the molar and the incisors for the canine teeth.

(e) The canine teeth between eighteen and twenty-four months of age.

(f) The four second molars, between twenty-four and thirty months of age.

If babies have received certain antibiotics early in life, their baby teeth may be stained brown. There is nothing the dentist can do about this. The permanent teeth, however, will not be discolored.

The first permanent teeth will appear at about six years of age and are already being formed after a few months of life. The first baby teeth lost are the lower, central incisors. They are lost in approximately the same order in which they came in. The permanent teeth that take the place of the baby molars are called bicuspids. The six year molars come in behind the baby molars and the twelve year molars behind the six year molars. Permanent teeth are usually completed by fourteen years of age. The eighteen year molars called wisdom teeth sometimes never come in.

Teeth Knocked Out—If any temporary teeth are knocked out they should be promptly reinserted in their sockets by the child's parents. Tooth replantation helps delay the use of a prosthetic device and avoids the psychological trauma of loss of the front teeth.

TEMPERATURE—FEVER

Our temperature is not always 98.6 degrees as most people believe. There is a normal variation every day. In children up to a year or two of age, 100 degrees is a normal temperature. A temperature of 101 degrees or more means that some type of illness is present.

Taking the temperature under the arm is unsatisfactory since it is not accurate enough. Feeling if the child is hot leaves too much room for error. Oral temperatures are difficult because children will not cooperate. Rectal temperatures are the best and most accurate. I explain how to take the temperature and read the thermometer under the heading "Thermometer—Rectal."

If your child has fever, taking the temperature every four hours while awake is sufficient, unless he should feel extremely hot or has had a previous febrile convulsion. If the fever has been low grade for a few days, once or twice a day is enough. The temperature will fluctuate in the course of most diseases. It may be high (104°) for a few days, then almost normal, and then go up again. This does not mean the child is better or worse. When children are sick they are prone to run a higher fever than adults. It is also possible to be quite sick without fever. I like to see a sick child run a fever. Then I know that one of his body's defensive mechanisms is at work fighting infection. Fever also lets the mother know that the child is sick and gives her some indication whether or not to consult the physician. Do not contact your doctor immediately after your child develops fever. It is too early to establish proper diagnosis. The disease process must have time to unfold and produce positive findings on physical examination in order for your physician to make a diagnosis. A physician will not start specific therapy until an exact diagnosis is established. If a child seen too early is examined, twenty-four hours later, it may be obvious that tonsillitis is present which requires specific antibiotic therapy. Thus, one trip to the doctor's office may have been unnecessary.

The important question is not the fever, but the other signs and symptoms present or developing. Parents must not be distracted from making more important observations. Occasionally, convulsions are precipitated by high fever, but this can usually be prevented by controlling the fever and sedating the child. Authorities agree that febrile convulsions rarely result in permanent brain damage. Prior to the advent of modern medicine, certain peculiar diseases were treated with heat to cause 107–108 degree fevers without damage to the brain. Since the testicles are located in the scrotum and therefore not affected by high fever, sterility is not a problem. (See Aspirin, Convulsions, Tempra, Tylenol.)

TEMPER TANTRUMS

All children have temper tantrums. They are particularly frequent before three years of age, because of the frustration children feel when they are not permitted to do as they please. Parents must not be controlled by temper tantrums. The young child in the grocery store may lie down in the middle of the floor and kick and scream. Let him do it. Ignore the temper tantrum to the best of your ability and go on about your business even though it is personally embarrassing. Temper tantrums represent non-specific behavior. When the child is older he will deal directly with the person that he has these angry feelings toward. However, frequent temper tantrums may be a sign of an emotional problem that requires counseling.

TEMPRA

Tempra is a safe and effective medication that is used for the relief of pain and control of fever. It is not a salicylate like aspirin. It contains no caffeine. It is particularly valuable for patients who do not tolerate aspirin well. It may also be used in conjunction with aspirin. It is identical with tylenol. Tempra is available in two forms —tempra *drops* and tempra *syrup*. It may be purchased in the drugstore without a prescription. The dosage of tempra *drops* is:

(a) Under one year of age, 0.6 of a cc, three to four times a day.

(b) One to three years of age, 0.6 of a cc to 1.2 cc's three to four times a day.

(c) Three to six years of age, 1.2 cc's three to four times a day.

(d) Six to twelve years of age, 2.4 cc's three to four times a day.

The dosage of tempra *syrup* is:

(a) Under one year of age one-half teaspoon three or four times a day.

(b) One to three years of age, one-half to one teaspoon three or four times a day.

(c) Three to six years of age, one teaspoon three or four times a day.

(d) Six to twelve years of age, two teaspoons three or four times a day.

TESTICLE—UNDESCENDED (CRYPTORCHIDISM)

In the newborn period the testicles are not always found in the scrotum. However, if they can be pushed down into the scrotum the baby's testicles will usually descend by themselves at a later date. A good way for the parents to determine if the testicles are really undescended is while they are bathing the infant in a tub of warm water. This relaxes the child and may be the only time it will be possible to feel the testicles in the scrotum. Then the parents and physician know everything is all right. Undescended testicles may involve one or both sides, but the latter is rare. A boy with one or even both testicles undescended will have all the normal secondary sex characteristics of males. If the testicle does not descend before the age of puberty, treatment is indicated as a testicle that remains undescended will not produce sperm for reproduction. Occasionally, hormone shots are helpful. If not, surgery is indicated. The results are excellent.

TETANUS (LOCKJAW)

Tetanus is an infectious disease that enters the body through dirty wounds.

A. Signs and Symptoms. For tetanus to develop, injury to the body must occur. The onset is gradual spasms of the neck and jaw and difficulty in swallowing. There is increased irritability, headache, chills, fever, and generalized pains followed by convulsions.

B. Etiology (Cause). Tetanus is caused by a product excreted by a specific bacteria called an exotoxin.

C. Treatment. The wound is cleaned and tetanus antitoxin injected around it. However, this may not be of much value once the disease process has started. Antibiotic is usually prescribed. The patient is kept in a quiet, dark room because minor stimulation may cause convulsions. Convulsions are controlled with appropriate sedatives. The outlook in spite of treatment is poor. The survival rate is approximately 50 per cent.

D. Incubation Period. The incubation period is one day to three weeks; usually eight to twelve days.

E. Prevention. The best treatment is adequate prevention. (See Immunizations.)

If an injury occurs at night or on the weekend that does not require your doctor's attention, *it is safe to wait for a tetanus booster* until his routine office hours. There is no emergency in receiving a tetanus booster.

THERMOMETER—RECTAL

All parents should buy a rectal thermometer and learn how to use it before their baby comes home from the hospital. Ask a relative, friend or the doctor's nurse to show you how. For those who want to try themselves, instructions are given below:

The bulb of a rectal thermometer contains mercury. The heat of the body expands this mercury and drives it along the shaft of the thermometer, which is calibrated in degrees. Before taking the temperature shake the thermometer down. This may be done by holding it firmly between your thumb and forefinger and vigorously shaking with a sharp snapping motion. The mercury should be shaken down to at least 97 degrees. If the mercury does not go down, you are not shaking the thermometer hard enough.

Before inserting the thermometer place vaseline on its tip (bulb). If vaseline is not available, use cold cream. The baby is best held on his stomach across your knees. The thermometer is then gently inserted into the rectum for approximately two inches. Push the thermometer gently and it will find its own course. Leave the thermometer in place for three minutes. In an older child, the temperature may be easily taken while he is lying on his side and his knees drawn up a little. It is too difficult to find the rectum when he is lying flat on his stomach.

Reading the thermometer is easy once you get the hang of it. Thermometers have one edge sharper than the other. This sharp edge should point towards you. In this position the marks for the temperature in degrees are above the mercury and the numbers below. Roll the thermometer very slightly in your hand until the light is such that you can see the column of mercury. Read the number at the end of the column of mercury. This is the child's temperature. The scale on a rectal thermometer is from 94 degrees to 106 degrees. If you get a reading at either extreme, look again. These extreme temperatures are not compatible with life. Do not be concerned too much over the fractions of a degree. It makes little difference to your doctor if the temperature is 98.6 or 98.8. The doctor is only interested in the approximate temperature. Be sure to tell your doctor how you took the temperature—that is rectally, or orally.

THRUSH

Thrush is a fungus infection involving the sides of the mouth, tongue and gums. It is not a sign of uncleanliness. Thrush is a common occurrence, particularly in the newborn. It looks like white patches of milk, but if an attempt is made to scrape the patches off, bleeding occurs. Gentian violet is used but this is quite messy and not too effective. Call your doctor during office hours so that he may prescribe antifungal drops to squirt on the involved area.

Thrush may also occur in the gastrointestinal tract after the prolonged use of antibiotics. Antibiotics kill the normal organisms in our gastrointestinal tract which allows the bowel to be over-run with the fungus. The stools become loose and diarrhea many develop. Often no specific treatment is necessary. Once the antibiotic is discontinued, the fungus will probably disappear. However, Lactinex is frequently prescribed. Lactinex Granules are a mixed culture of organisms that help establish speedy restoration of the normal intestinal flora. Be sure to keep this drug refrigerated. In addition, in stubborn cases follow the recommendation found under the treatment of diarrhea.

THUMB SUCKING

Sucking is a normal instinct. If your baby immediately starts to suck his thumb after each feeding, give him more time on the bottle or breast to satisfy this instinct. Do not confuse thumb sucking with the hand chewing that all babies do when teething begins.

Thumb sucking seems to be less common in breast fed babies. This is probably so because the baby gets a longer opportunity to suck since mother does not know exactly when her breast is empty. The bottle fed baby usually has the bottle taken away as it should be when it is empty.

As the baby gets stronger, and the nipple is worn out, he is able to feed more rapidly. To provide more time for sucking, as the infant does not enjoy sucking air, purchase new hard rubber nipples with small holes. However, it is not just the length of each feeding, but also the frequency of feeding that determines if the sucking instinct is satisfied.

Thumb sucking pushes the upper teeth forward and the lower teeth back. This has no effect on the permanent teeth. Mittens or restraints of any nature should not be used. This would only frustrate the baby and create anger on his part. Applying alum to the thumb does not break this habit either. Punishing the child or constantly reminding him to stop sucking the thumb seems to be of no value. If anything, it draws the child's attention to the problem and prolongs its duration. If the parents can divert the child's interest to something, it will usually stop the immediate problem. Chewing on a corner of a blanket or toy is equivalent to thumb sucking.

Thumb sucking in the older child is often a means of comforting himself. The child will suck his thumb when he is frustrated and overly tired. It helps put him to sleep. The child uses thumb sucking to retreat to a more infantile level of behavior. If the child between one and three years of age sucks his thumb occasionally during the day or at bedtime and seems normal in other respects, I would accept it as normal behavior. If thumb sucking occurs most of the day, the problem should be discussed with your physician to determine if there are any psychological problems present. Thumb sucking goes away spontaneously with time and is only a problem if it persists beyond the age of five. At this time it may affect the permanent teeth and, thus, the bite. I have seen dentists convince older children to stop sucking their thumbs—probably because they represent an outside authority figure.

TONGUE

A. Tongue Tied

The tongue is attached to the floor of the mouth by the frenulum, which is a piece of tissue that looks as if it were a piece of string. If the frenulum interferes with mobility of the tongue, the newborn baby may not be able to suck adequately. The infant is "tongue tied." Your physician solves this problem by cutting the frenulum with scissors in his office. If a child has gotten along without having his frenulum cut as an infant, it has nothing to do with poor speech or stuttering when he is older.

B. Geographic Tongue

The normal tongue occasionally resembles a contour map that changes configuration. These patterns on the tongue are no cause for alarm; no disease is present.

TONSILLITIS

Inflammation (infection) of the tonsils is called tonsillitis. The tonsils are normally large during the first five years of life, but usually shrink rapidly in size thereafter.

A. Signs and Symptoms. If the parents look into the back of the throat with a flashlight they may be able to see that the tonsils are swollen and red. White patches of pus may also be present. These are the same signs that your physician sees. Fever is not always present. Associated symptoms may include vomiting, abdominal cramping, sore throat, headache, and swollen glands in the neck.

B. Etiology (Cause). Many different viruses and bacteria cause tonsillitis.

C. Treatment. The treatment depends upon the cause. Antibiotic is of no value in a viral infection. If a bacterial infection is present your physician will choose the appropriate antibiotic based upon his clinical judgment. The recommendations given under the treatment of the common cold are most helpful.

D. Incubation. The incubation period depends upon the causitive organism.

E. Communicability. The communicability depends upon the organism causing the infection. If tonsillitis is caused by a streptococcus, it is highly communicable and all children in the same family should receive preventive penicillin therapy. (See Scarlet Fever and Strep Throat.)

F. School Attendance. School may be resumed with the approval of your physician or after the patient has been without fever for forty-eight hours and is feeling well.

G. Complications. Complications of tonsillitis are rare. Occasionally, an abscess will form behind the tonsils. This is called quinsy. This abscess must be surgically drained. After complete recovery removal of the tonsils is indicated. When tonsillitis is caused by a streptococcal infection, and is not treated for ten to fourteen days with appropriate antibiotic therapy, nephritis and rheumatic fever may occur. (See Nephritis, Rheumatic Fever.)

H. Indications for Removal of Tonsils. Many parents after one attack of tonsillitis ask if it is necessary to have the tonsils removed. The answer is "no." There are four indications for removing the tonsils.

1. Repeated attacks of tonsillitis which most physicans define as six or more attacks per year.
2. Enlarged tonsils that obstruct the airway and interfere with breathing.
3. Enlarged tonsils that interfere with the quality of speech.
4. After complete recovery from a tonsillar abscess.

The operation is not advised for repeated colds, chronic cough or loss of appetite. Tonsillectomy was more frequently preformed prior to modern antibiotic therapy. *Since the advent of antibiotics I believe that too many tonsils are being taken out without proper medical justification.* No operation is simple. Complications are always possible. *Anytime a child must be put to sleep for an operation I have the utmost respect for the procedure.*

A deep level of anesthesia is necessary to remove the tonsils. Therefore, physicians prefer to wait until the child is four years of age before operating, except under special circumstances. The parent is doing his child a disservice if he pressures the doctor to remove the tonsils. It is true that the child would not have any more attacks of tonsillitis, but that doesn't mean there will be a magical improvement in his health. Infections may occur elsewhere in the body more frequently.

Post-Operative Instructions. If your child has had his tonsils and adenoids removed, his physician will give you, the parents, post-operative instructions that he wants you to follow at home. Post-operatively, throat secretions may be a little thick and there may be some mouth odor noticed. Strong efforts to clear the throat and gargling should be discouraged. Increasing the amount of fluid taken will help keep secretions as loose as possible. Changes in speech, including a nasal quality to the voice, is common after surgery. However, these changes should disappear in a few weeks. It is usually advisable for the child to stay in bed for two days after discharge from the hospital. Keep the child indoors for the remainder of the first week and do not let him engage in strenuous

289

play or get over-heated. A liquid diet is indicated for the first two or three days until the child wants to progress to a soft diet. Citrus juices usually sting the back of the throat so they should be avoided. Milk, soft drinks, ice cream, and Jell-O are fine to give after surgery. Do not eat toast or hard rolls, which might scratch the throat, until after the first week. Throat discomfort and referred ear pain are to be expected. Aspirin and tempra or tylenol are indicated. (See respective headings.) Chewing gum helps keep the throat muscles relaxed and moist. The operating surgeon should be *called immediately* under the following circumstances:

1. Vomiting of fresh or old blood.
2. Constant ear pain.
3. Temperature greater than 102 degrees.
4. Unusually dark bowel movements—this may represent blood in the stool.

TRACHEITIS

The air we breathe in is carried into our chest by a large tube called the trachea, which then subdivides into large and small bronchi that go to our lungs. Tracheitis means that the trachea is infected.

A. Signs and Symptoms. The signs and symptoms may include a previous history of a cold, a cough that is often worse at night and first thing in the morning, hoarseness, low grade fever, and swollen glands in the neck.

B. Etiology (Cause). Tracheitis may be either a viral or bacterial infection. Some cases are allergic in origin.

C. Treatment. The treatment depends upon the cause. Antibiotic is of no value in a viral infection. If a bacterial infection is present, your physician will choose the appropriate antibiotic based upon his clinical judgment. Antihistamines may be helpful along with a cough syrup. A vaporizer is sometimes of value. If on an allergic basis, steroids (cortisone) may be necessary. The recommendations given under the treatment of the common cold are helpful.

D. Incubation Period. The incubation period depends upon the cause.

E. Communicability. Tracheitis is not highly communicable.

F. School Attendance.   School should not be attended until the signs and symptoms have disappeared or permission has been given by the child's physician.

G. Complications.   The infection may spread lower in the respiratory tree, causing bronchitis or pneumonia.

TUBERCULOSIS

It is important to have a certain philosophy about tuberculosis. The disease must be considered or the diagnosis will be missed. A person can have tuberculosis and feel well. Fifty thousand new active cases are occurring yearly.

Tuberculosis is no longer the dread disease it was years ago. Adequate means of treatment are available with medications which were not previously in use. The advent of modern surgical techniques has also added new weapons with which to fight this disease. Just about everybody in his lifetime develops tuberculosis. In the vast majority of cases, however, the person develops resistance to tuberculosis, throws it off, and never knows he was ill.

Tuberculosis is not inherited, it is communicated from person to person, mostly through the air. Adequate means of case finding are available through your local health department.

I am not using the format developed in the presentation of other infectious illnesses, since tuberculosis may mimic any other disease and may involve any body system. Tuberculosis in children is entirely different than tuberculosis in adults. In adults most people are used to thinking of a cavity in the lungs, weight loss, loss of appetite, fatigue, spitting up of sputum, and fever. Any child who has a persistent cough which does not respond to the usual medication may have tuberculosis. A chest X ray is advisable under these circumstances. All cases of tuberculosis are reported to the health department which investigates all contacts. If there is a case of tuberculosis in your family, or if it is suspected, chest X rays at regular intervals are usually done by the health department. I recommend that all household help have an X ray of their chests as a condition of employment. Every child of preschool age should have a yearly tuberculin skin test.

Tuberculosis was commonly tested for by means of a patch on the back between the shoulder blades, but an easier way is by use of the Tine Test. With this test, four little puncture marks are made in the skin of the forearm. The test is read for any hardness (induration, lump) after forty-eight and seventy-two hours. Redness without hardness is a negative test. If a child develops a positive skin test to tuberculosis, it does not mean that he has active disease. It simply means that he has tuberculosis germs in his body. Most children develop what is called a primary complex in the lung and never know they resisted tuberculosis by themselves. However, children under three or four years of age that develop a positive skin test to tuberculosis should be given prophylactic medication. INH and PAS are commonly used. These drugs are prescribed by your physician to prevent the complication of tubercular meningitis which commonly occurs in young children. This preventive medication is given for a minimum of one year. It is frequently provided free of charge by the health department. The child will also be followed with chest X rays at appropriate intervals.

Tuberculosis can be cured today, but the earlier treatment is started the better. A special climate is no longer considered important. A complete cure takes two to five years. Popular medications used in the treatment of active tuberculosis consist of streptomycin, PAS and INH. Ethamyanbutal, a new oral antituberculosis drug, effective against strains of the tubercle bacillus, resistant to previous known agents, has been recently added to your physician's armamentarium.

Bacillus, Calmette-Guerin is available for children who have negative tuberculin tests and cannot avoid having contact with tuberculosis. This vaccine is composed of pig tubercle bacilli whose potency has been reduced by special cultural procedures. The administration of the vaccine to man produces a harmless infection which establishes a limited immunity to reinfection with tubercle bacilli of man. Although there have been many doubts concerning the immediate safety of the vaccine, there is no evidence that tubercular disease, other than the lesion of inoculation, has resulted from its use. The vaccine may be administered to anyone who has a negative skin test for tuberculosis. It is given by injection. In the United States the indications for the use of BCG are questionable. In many areas of the world where tuberculosis is commonly associated with a high death rate, vaccination programs have been undertaken. Such programs have been sponsored by the World Health Organization, and proven very successful.

TYLENOL

Tylenol is a safe and effective medication that is used for the relief of pain and control of fever. It is not a salicylate like aspirin. It contains no caffeine. It is particularly valuable for patients who do not tolerate aspirin well. It may be used in conjunction with aspirin to control high fever, or by itself. It is identical to tempra. Tylenol is available in three forms. It may be purchased in the drugstore without a prescription. The dosage of tylenol *drops* is:

(a) Under one year of age, 0.6 of a cc three or four times a day.
(b) One to three years of age, 0.6 of a cc to 1.2 cc's three or four times a day.
(c) Three to six years of age, 1.2 cc's three to four times a day.

The dosage of *elixir* of tylenol is:

(a) Under one year of age, one-half teaspoon three or four times a day.
(b) One to three years of age, one-half to one teaspoon three or four times a day.
(c) Three to six years of age, one teaspoon three or four times a day.
(d) Over six years of age, two teaspoons three or four times a day.

Tylenol *tablets* may also be used for children six to twelve years of age.

One-half to one tablet three or four times a day.

TYPHOID FEVER

Typhoid fever is an infectious disease usually induced through food or drink.

A. Signs and Symptoms. The characteristic sign and symptom is fluctuating fever. Interestingly enough, the fever is associated with a slow pulse. A typical rash called "rose spots" may appear at the end of the first week. This rash usually occurs over the back and abdomen (belly). The spleen frequently becomes enlarged. The diagnosis is confirmed by obtaining adequate cultures and isolating the organism. Special blood tests become positive after the first week of illness.

B. Etiology (Cause).   A specific bacteria transmitted by water, milk and food contaminated by active cases or carriers. Typhoid may also be transmitted indirectly by flies.

C. Treatment.   Specific antibiotic therapy is available. The duration of treatment is determined by the patient's general response. Particular attention is paid to the control of fever.

D. Incubation.   The incubation period is seven to fourteen days.

E. Period of Communicability.   The patient is communicable as long as the specific bacteria may be isolated from his stools.

F. School Attendance.   School attendance should not be permitted until at least three consecutive negative stool cultures are obtained.

G. Prevention.   Modern sanitation plays a major role in preventing typhoid fever. (See Immunizations.)
able to completely eradicate the specific causative organism, thus

H. Complications.   The main problem is that of not being
leading to a carrier state. This is why health cards are mandatory
the story of "Typhoid Mary." Intestinal rupture is a rare compli-
for all people in the food industry. I am sure that everyone recalls
cation that requires surgical repair.

U

ULCER—PEPTIC

Peptic ulcer in children is more common than most people believe. Many cases are discovered when a child has a complete workup for recurrent belly pain. Ulcer pain is recurrent in nature and usually relieved by food. In children the pain is frequently located around the navel. Weight loss, which is a major symptom in adults, may not occur. The diagnosis is proven by X ray. Diets consisting of large amounts of milk and cream, antacids and relaxants for the gastrointestinal tract are used as they are in adults. In addition, *it is mandatory that all children with ulcers have psychological testing and psychotherapy.* I do not believe that a permanent cure can be effected without taking into consideration the emotional aspects which seem to be the overwhelming cause of ulcers in children. An example of a typical ulcer diet is as follows:

First Week

3 oz. (6 tbl.) whole milk and 1 oz. (2 tbl.) cream are to be taken every hour from 7 a.m. to 9 p.m., or later if necessary. Additions are made to the diet as follows:

	Breakfast	Midmorning	Dinner	Midafternoon	Supper	Bedtime
1st and 2nd days	Only the 4 oz. milk and cream is taken every hour from 7 a.m. to 9 p.m.					
3rd thru 7th day		Sieved cereal	Soft cooked or poached egg or custard or raw egg mixed with milk		Sieved cereal or custard or egg as at dinner. Cocoa (¼ tsp. cocoa, ¾ cup milk, ¼ cup cream and a little sugar)	

Second Week

Continue the milk and cream mixture every hour.

	Breakfast	Midmorning	Dinner	Midafternoon	Supper	Bedtime
8th, 9th and 10th days	Sieved cereal	Soda crackers or white toast	Soft-cooked or poached egg or custard. Baked potato (no skin) or mashed potato.	Custard or Jell-O or plain tapioca pudding or other plain pudding	Sieved cereal or custard or eggs as at dinner. White toast or milk toast. Cocoa as above.	

Second Week (continued)

	Breakfast	Midmorning	Dinner	Midafternoon	Supper	Bedtime
11th thru 14th day	Sieved cereal	Soda crackers or white toast	Soft-cooked or poached egg or custard, baked potato (no skin) or mashed potato or rice—white toast	Custard or Jell-O or plain tapioca pudding or other plain pudding	Cream soup made with sieved vegetables, soda crackers, Junket or soft custard or simple pudding or sieved applesauce, cocoa as above	

CEREALS TO USE: Strained oatmeal, farina, cream of wheat, grits. Only a very small amount of sugar and salt should be used. No pepper. Toast and potatoes may be buttered. Four ounces of milk and cream if the patient awakens during the night.

Third Week

Discontinue the milk and cream mixture every hour. Instead, use only the foods at the time indicated.

	Breakfast	Midmorning	Dinner	Midafternoon	Supper	Bedtime
15th 16th and 17th days	Sieved cereal, soft-cooked or poached egg, white toast, ½ glass milk and cream or cocoa (¼ tsp. cocoa-¾ cup	Soda crackers or white toast, ½ glass milk and cream	½ serving canned strained beef, veal or liver or well ground meat (no pork or ham), or cream of vegetable soup, or soft-cooked or	Custard or Jell-O or plain tapioca pudding or other plain pudding or vanilla ice cream, ½ cream, ½	Sieved cereal or plain boiled rice or cottage or cream cheese or egg as at breakfast, white toast, plain Jell-O or	1 glass milk and cream

Third Week (continued)

	Breakfast	Midmorning	Dinner	Midafternoon	Supper	Bedtime
	milk-¼ cup cream and a little sugar)		poached egg, baked potato (no skin), or mashed potato or rice, sieved vegetable, if not used in soup. White toast or soda crackers, ½ glass milk and cream	glass milk and cream	sieved fruit or baked apple without seeds or peel or very ripe banana or vanilla ice cream, ½ glass milk and cream, ½ glass strained orange juice diluted with water, at end of meal	
18th thru 21st days	Same as Above	Same as Above	Same as Above Plain pudding or Jell-O or vanilla ice cream	Same as Above	Same as Above Sieved vegetable	Same as Above

VEGETABLES TO USE: Sieved asparagus, beets, carrots, English peas, green beans, greens, spinach and squash. Toast and vegetables may be buttered. Only a small amount of salt and sugar should be used. No pepper. ½ glass of milk and cream if the patient awakens during the night.

22nd day on: Use convalescent ulcer or bland diet. Usually the patient should stay on the bland diet (with nourishments at midmorning, midafternoon and bedtime) for at least six months.

Bland or Convalescent Ulcer Diet

Approximately: 2300 calories
230 grams carbohydrates
120 grams protein
100 grams fat

It omits highly seasoned foods, gas forming foods and foods high in roughage. Foods should be served warm or cool, never hot or cold.

SERVE EVERY DAY	DO NOT SERVE
1. MILK: 1 quart or more—whole pasteurized, or preferably homogenized milk. May be used as a beverage or in cooked food. Buttermilk, milk drinks, cocoa, eggnog, milk shake, cocoamalt, Ovaltine, evaporated milk.	
2. EGG: 1 or more	Fried or hard cooked eggs.
3. MEAT OR ALTERNATE: 2 servings or more. Beef, lamb, veal, fish or poultry. Meats should be ground if they are not tender and should be served without gravy or rich sauces. Canned salmon or tuna, canned chopped meats for junior. Creamed meats, crisp bacon, cottage, cream or mild American cheese. Small amount of smooth peanut butter.	Fried meats. Frankfurters, bologna, luncheon meats, sausage, pork products, except bacon. Strongly flavored cheese.
4. POTATO OR ALTERNATE: 1 serving or more white potato. Hominy, macaroni, noodles, rice or spaghetti may be served occasionally.	Fried potato, potato chips.
5. VEGETABLES: 2 servings or more, cooked green beans, wax beans, asparagus tips, beets, carrots, young English peas, lima beans, spinach, milk flavored greens, pumpkin, squash (without skins or seeds). If vegetables are not young and tender, they must be sieved. Raw tender chopped lettuce.	Raw vegetables except for tender chopped lettuce. Turnips, cabbage, corn, dried beans, dried peas, onions, and any other not listed.
6. FRUIT: 2 servings or more. One serving should be ½ cup (4 ozs.) strained orange juice or grapefruit juice as part of a meal (not between meals). Other strained juices, ripe banana or grapefruit or orange section. Canned or cooked apples, pears, peaches, white cherries or apricots, all without skins or seeds.	Any other except avocado.
7. BREAD: 3 servings or more. White, fine whole wheat or rye bread without seeds, hard rolls or soda crackers. Spoon bread.	Hot breads as corn bread, biscuits, pancakes, bran rolls, coarse dark breads. Cracked wheat bread.

SERVE EVERY DAY	DO NOT SERVE
8. CEREAL: 1 serving. Cooked cereals such as farina, cream of wheat, infant cereals, strained oatmeal and pettijohns. Dry cereals such as corn flakes, rice krispies, puffed rice and puffed wheat.	Bran flakes, all bran, cracked wheat and other coarse cereals.
9. FAT: 3 squares or more margarine or butter. Cream may be served as desired.	Fried foods, gravies, any other.
10. SOUP: Cream soups made with vegetables allowed. Oyster stew.	Other cream soups, meat broth should not be served to ulcer patient.
11. DESSERT: Custard, pudding, ice cream, sherbet and ices without fruit or nuts, plain cookies, cake without fruit or nuts, Jell-O, sweet sauces without nuts, coarse fruits or seeds.	Pies and other pastries, cake with dried fruit or nuts.
12. SWEETS: Sugar, honey, syrup, jelly, molasses or plain candy in moderation.	Jam, marmalade.
13. Beverage: Milk, cream and weak tea.	Strong tea. Soft drinks.
14. MISCELLANEOUS: Salt in reasonable amounts. Cream sauce.	Spices, nuts, coffee, cocoanut, olives, pickles, pepper.

URINE (COLOR)

The color of the urine is determined by what the child eats, and by his total fluid intake. Many parents are concerned if the urine becomes dark when the child is sick. There is no cause for alarm. The child is excreting the same amount of waste products. The urine is just more concentrated. Red urine should always be significant to the parents as blood may be present. (See Nephritis.) Occasionally, the eating of beets will cause the urine to appear red, but sensible parents should check with their physician.

V

VAGINAL BLEEDING

Vaginal bleeding may be due to:

1. A foreign body in the vagina.

2. Menstruation if the child is at the age of puberty.
3. A withdrawal reaction in the newborn from the maternal female hormones.

(See Foreign Objects, Newborn—Vagina.)

VAGINAL DISCHARGE (VAGINITIS)

Vaginitis in young girls is very common. Before the age of puberty the mucous membrane of the vagina has not been affected by the female hormone estrogen which makes the mucous membrane tougher and, therefore, more able to resist infection. The anatomy of this region is such that the vagina can easily become contaminated with stool or urine, thus leading to infection. These non-specific infections respond well to vinegar douches four times a day. Mix one tablespoon of vinegar with a quart of water. Sit your child in a basin or tub and splash this mixture into the vagina. If the discharge lasts for more than a few days, consult your physician. A foreign object placed in the vagina is always a possibility.

VITAMINS

Vitamins are recommended routinely for children under a year of age. There are hundreds of multivitamin preparations on the market with or without fluoride. Any of the multivitamin preparations which contain fluoride are satisfactory. Fluoride is strongly recommended because it reduces the incidence of tooth decay. However, if your town should be fortunate enough to have fluoride occurring naturally or added to the water supply, multivitamins without fluoride are recommended. A prescription is necessary for vitamins containing fluoride. This appears ridiculous to me since fluoride will not hurt you. However, since this is the law contact your physician during regular office hours. Most physicans recommend vitamins in drop form. The dosage is 0.3 cc's every day for infants less than six months of age, and 0.6 cc's every day for infants between six months and one year of age. The time of day vitamins are given makes little difference, but it is best to establish some pattern. The already prepared formulas such as Similac, Enfamil, etc., have vitamins added to them; therefore, only supple-

300

mental fluoride drops are necessary. The usual recommended dosage is one-half cc every day.

The use of vitamins in the United States has become almost a fetish and is vastly overdone. Too many vitamins are sold and taken unnecessarily. Nutritional disease due to an inadequate and incorrect food intake was prevalent years ago, but has vanished wherever medical knowledge has been linked with adequate availability and proper administration of food. It seems impossible to develop a vitamin deficiency if you eat a normal diet. If additional vitamins are indicated after the first year of life, children will probably prefer the soft chewable tablets. One a day is sufficient.

VOMITING IN INFANCY (SPITTING) (ALSO SEE GASTRITIS)

Many infants will naturally spit up a great deal, or occasionally vomit everything for no apparent reason after feedings. This is perfectly normal and is to be expected. An annoying type of vomiting or spitting up may occur for months in active, healthy, vigorous babies who gain weight and develop normally. If the formula contains butterfat, the odor of sour vomitus often permeates the house. Fortunately, vomiting of this nature usually stops when the baby learns to sit up at about six months of age. There is no specific treatment. The parents should be reassured by the normal growth and development of their infant.

Children, when they are angry, can deliberately vomit. They will do this if they see that it gains them attention. Parents simply cannot let themselves be controlled by this type of behavior. If the child is in bed the parents might have to let him stay in the vomitus and clean it up when he is asleep.

The common causes of vomiting in infancy that need treatment are:

1. Any disease process associated with fever. Vomiting is usually marked only at the onset of such a disease, but may persist as long as the fever.
2. Excessive food may cause over-distention of the stomach and thus vomiting.
3. Indigestion from improperly prepared formulas or food.
4. Intestinal allergy.

301

5. Intestinal obstruction. The vomiting is forceful or projectible in nature. (See Intestinal Obstruction.)

6. Increased pressure in the central nervous system such as might occur in hydrocephalus or brain hemorrhage.

7. Psychological factors such as a tense, nervous mother.

8. Environmental factors such as handling the baby too much.

WALKING AND SHOES

No baby, when he begins to walk, walks like a normal adult. The baby will either turn his feet in, turn his feet out, or walk on the outside or inside of the soles of his feet. Often the knees will be knocked. All these minor variations correct themselves with time and should be of no concern to the parent. (See Growth and Development, Knocked Knees.)

If shoes are put on too early, they may impede the baby's ability to walk. They are not necessary until the child is walking alone since shoes are for the protection of the feet. Even then it is good for the person to go barefooted in the house. Improper shoes may cause foot deformities during the first three years of life. Inexpensive tiny fashionable shoes are available, but they are bad for the feet. The dogma of positive support for the feet is no longer tenable.

Most parents ask for specific suggestions regarding shoes. I recommend the "Wikler Shoes" manufactured by the Brown Shoe Company. Any store that sells Buster Brown Shoes will have them. This shoe was specially designed by Simon J. Wikler, a podiatrist, to prevent foot deformities from developing. The shoe is more or less squared off in the front so that the toes are not squeezed together. The growing foot will not be constricted, and the child will be able to use all his foot muscles.

WARTS (VERRUCA)

The exact cause of warts is unknown. Most physicians believe they are caused by a virus. Very small warts need no treatment. Larger warts (1/8") should be removed if they are subject to ir-

302

ritation, and may be removed for cosmetic reasons. The most popular treatments are the application of medicine or dry ice, electrocautery, and surgical excision. Regardless of the treatment chosen, warts are apt to recur. It is interesting to note that warts sometimes disappear spontaneously.

WEIGHT GAIN—BABY'S

The average baby seen in private practice gains approximately a pound and a half a month. Some babies will gain only a pound a month and others two pounds. These are perfectly normal variations. The amount of weight the baby gains will depend somewhat upon his original birth weight. The average baby at birth weighs approximately seven and one-half pounds. He doubles his birth weight by six months of age and triples it at a year. It is obvious therefore that the rate at which weight is gained as the baby grows older slows down. Weight gain cannot be taken as an isolated factor. It must be correlated with the baby's general health and growth and development. *Too many mothers state that their baby doesn't eat enough, but this is impossible when the weight gain is normal.* Obviously, the baby must be eating enough food to satisfy his need.

WELL BABY VISITS—FIRST YEAR OF LIFE

Every baby should have a physical examination once a month during the first year of life. This is a very important part of preventive pediatrics.

The doctor, at each well-baby visit, will weigh and measure the baby. He will measure the circumference of the baby's head and chest and observe his growth and development carefully. The baby will be completely undressed and thoroughly examined. Congenital dislocation of the hips will be checked by placing the lower extremities in a frog-like position. (See Hip-Congenital Dislocation.) Crossed eyes will be looked for. (See Eyes.) Is an abdominal mass present? (See Wilm's Tumor.) These potentially serious problems can often be adequately treated with early diagnosis. This is one of the many advantages of routine well-baby visits.

All routine immunizations will be given and the doctor will discuss with the parents any problems that may arise. Parents should not feel embarrassed about asking questions. Any question that is asked is a sign of intelligence and shows your interest. Do not expect the doctor to be a mind reader. It is impossible for him to guess what your problems may be. Be brave and ask. The doctor will respect you more.

WHOOPING COUGH (PERTUSSIS)

Whooping cough refers to a characteristic sound, accompanying the deep intake of air following a series of coughs.

A. Signs and Symptoms. The early signs and symptoms are similar to a bad cold, with sneezing and coughing. Sometime later anywhere from a few days to two weeks, the characteristic whoop begins. Various degrees of cyanosis (blueness) of the lips may occur during the paroxysms of coughing. At the end of the explosive coughing efforts, vomiting often occurs, or the patient may swallow large amounts of thick mucous. The paroxysms of coughing are often initiated by eating, inhalation of smoke or sudden changes in temperature. The characteristic whoop is frequently absent in infants under one year of age. Laboratory tests are diagnostic in many cases. All suspected cases of whooping cough should be seen by the doctor.

B. Etiology (Cause). This disease is caused by a specific bacteria.

C. Treatment. Infants must be treated vigorously because the death rate is high. Hospitalization is indicated. An infant should be placed in a tent with oxygen and humidity. Specific antibiotic is available. Hyperimmune human serum once a day for two or three days is often of great value. Hyperimmune human serum is made from the blood of patients who recently recovered from whooping cough and developed a high antibody level that enabled them to fight this disease. Special nursing care is important to maintain a clear airway and prevent the aspiration of vomitus.

D. Incubation. The incubation period may be seven to twenty-one days, but ten days is most common.

E. Period of Communicability. This is during the cold period and the first three weeks of the whoop.

F. School Attendance. The patient is to be isolated for three weeks after the whoop is first heard. Other children in the family

304

may attend school, but should be closely observed by the teacher and barred from school immediately at the first sign of illness.

G. Prevention.   (See Immunizations.)

H. Complications.   The main complication in the young child is pneumonia which is associated with a high mortality rate.

WILM'S TUMOR

During the first year of life cancer is the leading cause of death in children. Wilm's tumor is one of the commonest forms. This tumor involves the kidney. The earliest means of making the diagnosis is at well-baby checkups when your physician feels the baby's abdomen (belly). A mass is almost always felt if a tumor is present. By the time the mother accidently feels such a mass while bathing the child, it is usually too late to effect a cure. If diagnosed early enough, a cure is possible. The diagnosis can be pretty well confirmed by X rays of the kidney. Treatment consists of removing the involved kidney, radiation, and anticancer drugs. Occasionally, the tumor will spread to the lungs.

General Index

A

Abdomen, 35
Abdominal distention, 79
Abdominal mass, 217
Abdominal pain, 35, 41, 46, 69, 98,
   141, 153, 195, 202, 211, 212,
   234, 274, 294
Abdominal pain, right lower part of
   abdomen, 46
Ability to read, 132
Abortion, therapeutic, 160
Abscesses, 33, 288
Abscesses, boils, carbuncles, 33
   furuncle, 33
   signs of infection, 33
      heat, 33
      pain, 33
      swelling, 33
      tenderness, 33
Abscesses, lung, 238
Accelerated growth, 184
Accidental swallowing of corrosive
      substance, chemical injury, 33
   acid, 33
   alkalies, 33
   esophagus, 33
   esophagus stricture, 34
   stomach, 33
Accidents, 51
Ace test tablets, 126
Acetone, 121
Acetone test, positive, 126
Acid, 33
Acidosis, 34
   bicarbonate, 34
   causes, 34
      aspirin poisoning, 34

Acidosis (*cont.*)
      diabetes, 34
      diarrhea, 34
      nephritis, 34
      starvation, 34
   signs and symptoms, 34
      dehydration, 34
         dry mouth, 34
         eyes, sunken, 34
         loss skin turgor, 34
         urination, decreased, 34
         weight loss, 34
      drowsiness, 34
      panting, 34
      restlessness, 34
Acidosis, diabetic, 121
Acne, 233
Acute appendicitis, 35
Adenitis, 35, 279
Adenoiditis, 36
Adenoids, 36, 134
Adrenalin, 58
Air conditioning, 58, 61
Air conditioning and colds, 95
Air conditioning filters, 61
Air conditioning, tax deduction, 58
Airplane sickness, 211
Albumin, 216
Alcohol-ear, 136
Alcohol-poisoning, 239
Alkali, 33
Allergic bronchitis, 65
Allergic nose, perennial allergic
      diagnosis, 38
   rhinitis (PAR), hayfever, 38
   signs and symptoms, 38
   treatment, 38
      antihistamine, 38

Cryptorchidism, 284
Cultures, 42
Cup, using, 166
Cure, asthma, 53
Curtains, for the asthmatic, 56
Cutaneous larva migrans, 108
Cuts, first aid for, 112
  control of bleeding, 112
    artery, 112
    tourniquet, 112
      releasing, 112
    vein, 112
  secondary infection, 113
  stitches, 112
  tendons, 112
  treatment, 112
    bandages, 112
    iodine, 112
    merthiolate, 112
    phisohex, 112
    tetanus booster, 112
Cyanosis (blueness), 101, 139
Cyst, Pilonidal, 232
Cystic fibrosis, 52, 107, 113
  allergies, associated, 115
  diagnosis, 114
    sweat test, 114
  etiology, 114
  life expectancy, 115
  signs and symptoms, 113
    chronic lung disease, 113
    distention of the abdomen, 114
    failure to gain weight, 114
    intestinal obstruction, 114
    pancreatic insufficiency, 114
    rectal prolapse, 114
    sweating, 113
  treatment, 115
    control of nutrition, 115
    control of pulmonary obstruc-
      tion, 115
    control of secondary pulmo-
      nary infection, 115
    correction of pancreatic insuf-
      ficiency, 115
Cystitis, 115, 183
  cystoscopic exam, 66
  diagnosis, 116
  etiology, 116

Cystitis (*cont.*)
  follow up, 117
  signs and symptoms, 116
    abdominal cramps, 116
    frequency of urination, 116
    pain in lower back, 116
    pain on urination, 116
    urgency, 116
  treatment, 116

D

Dark room, 206
DDT, 204
Deaf and dumb, 171
Debrox, 136
Decreased exercise tolerance, 101
Decreased urination, 34
Dehydration, 34,131,159
Delayed development of the teeth,
  186
Delirium, 202
Demand feeding, 148
Denco acetone powder, 126
Denial, 244
Denise-Browne splint, 88
Denver Development Screening
  test, 162
Depression of chest, 229
Desenex, 66
Desensitization, 37,39,198
  how long, 64
Desitin, 128
Detergents, 239
Development, 162
Diabetes, 34, 172
  coma and convulsions, 121
    Coca Cola, 121
  diet, 120
  foot care, 126
  heredity characteristics, 118
  hypoglycemia, 121
    diabetic acidosis, 121
    diabetic coma, 121
  incidence, 118
  injections, how to, 119
  insulin, 118
    globulin insulin, 119

315